THE 10 minute MENOPAUSE PLAN

Simple Daily Techniques for
HORMONAL BALANCE, ENERGY & HEALTHY EATING.

Linda Callen

Table of Contents

Introduction

———

"I didn't expect menopause to feel like this."

Linda Callen

———

For years, I thought I was prepared. I had always taken care of myself, eaten well, and kept moving. But when the hot flashes, brain fog, and bone-deep fatigue crept in, I felt blindsided. Suddenly, my body didn't respond the way it used to. I could push through a workout or tighten up my eating plan, but the results weren't the same. My moods were unpredictable. My memory felt unreliable. And underneath it all was a quiet fear: *Was this the new normal?*

I share this because I know I'm not alone. Many women describe this transition as disorienting, exhausting, even isolating. We've spent so much of our lives caring for others—children, partners, aging parents, and communities—that when our own needs start shouting at us, we're not sure how to respond.

My journey through menopause has been about listening. Listening to the signals my body was sending. Listening to the science about how our hormones shift in midlife. And listening to other women who were also searching for clarity, compassion, and practical strategies.

That's why I wrote this book. I want you to know that there *are* simple, effective ways to reclaim your energy, improve your mood, and feel like yourself again. You don't have to overhaul your whole life or chase impossible standards. Instead, you can begin with small, sustainable steps in just ten minutes at a time.

This book is not about perfection. It's about progress. It's about finding what works for *your* body in this season of life. It's about replacing confusion with confidence, and frustration with hope.

If you've ever thought, "I just want to feel normal again," you're in the right place. My goal is to walk alongside you with practical tools, gentle encouragement, and the reassurance that you are not broken. You are simply in transition and with the right care, this transition can become a time of renewal, strength, and even joy.

Let's begin, together.

Chapter 1

Hormonal Recalibration

———

"Your body isn't betraying you.
It's asking you to listen differently."

Lara Briden, *Hormone Repair Manual*

———

If you struggle to keep up with daily life the way you used to, you're not alone. Many women describe the transition into menopause as confusing and exhausting. You might feel tired, forgetful, emotional, out of shape, bloated, heavy, or sore. All of these symptoms are common and real.

This book will help you understand the science behind how your hormones and metabolism are changing. It will also help you make sense of the subtle recalibration happening throughout your body. Wisdom brings power. With the right knowledge and practical tools, you can adapt and start to feel like yourself again.

As you move through perimenopause and menopause, estrogen levels decline. This shift affects many systems in your body, not only reproduction. Every cell has estrogen receptors. Estrogen even influences the brain's control of mood and memory, which is why brain fog or emotional swings are common.

Estrogen has supported your mood, metabolism, muscles, bones, and brain since adolescence. Now, as it declines, your body naturally resets its rhythms. Progesterone also shifts, while hormones like thyroid, cortisol, and insulin become more prominent. These changes can feel unfamiliar. If you're unsure how to navigate this stage, this guide will walk you through the essentials: nutrition, exercise, sleep, and mindfulness practices that bring balance.

Carla, 52, had always been patient, focused, and easygoing. She worked with kids and usually had energy to spare at the end of the day. During menopause, things changed. She became more irritable and impatient, and by evening she felt forgetful and short-tempered. To cope, Carla began exercising with a friend twice a week. The routine cleared her head, boosted her mood, and gave her energy before dinner. It made a big difference, restoring harmony in her work and home life.

This book is here to guide you as you figure out what your body needs. The goal is to feel balanced, energized, and at peace, even during change. With patience and curiosity, you can explore your symptoms and discover new ways to care for yourself. Over time, you'll find more ease in daily life. Feel steadier. Sleep deeper. Move freer. One day at a time.

Restorative Habits

Rest is not a reward. It's a biological necessity.
Dr. Saundra Dalton-Smith, Sacred Rest

Your body is finding a new kind of balance. This shift affects brain function, mood, heart health, stress regulation, and even your immune system. Falling estrogen also slows metabolism and increases fat storage, especially around the abdomen. This change can raise your risk for cardiovascular disease, cancer, and stroke.

These risks remind us that the body now needs more care and attention to function well. You may notice signals, both subtle and obvious, long before you understand just how much has changed.

Hormone harmony isn't found. It's built. As Lara Briden explains in *The Hormone Repair Manual*, "Menopause is not a disease. It's a planned change, built into your biology. And it comes with new stability, resilience, and strength if you give your body what it needs." Many women feel frustrated when diet or exercise tweaks no longer work as quickly as before. The body processes carbs differently. It holds onto fat more easily. Intense workouts can raise cortisol instead of burning fat. Even dieting can slow metabolism further. Moderation works better here. Dr. Gabrielle Lyon, in *Forever Strong*, notes: "What got you here won't get you there. To thrive post-40, you need to prioritize muscle, not just weight loss."

Old advice like "eat less, and move more" misses the unique hormonal and metabolic demands of midlife. When your system is taxed, pushing harder drains more than it delivers. As Dr. Sara Gottfried says in *The Hormone Cure*, "What used to work now wears you down because the hormonal terrain has shifted." The new rules?

Think nourishment, not deprivation.

✦

Think strength, not size. Think support, not hustle.

Listen to what your body is asking for. Often, it's rest. Recovery-focused habits lower cortisol, support hormone balance, and build lasting energy. Try prioritizing practices like high-quality sleep, gentle movement (walking, yoga, or strength training), protein-rich meals, and mindfulness (breathwork, meditation, stretching). These simple steps calm the nervous system and restore balance.

The most effective strategies meet your body where it is. In midlife, recovery is essential. Making space for it expands your capacity to handle everything else in life. This guide emphasizes small, steady changes: 10-minute habits that compound over time, like interest in your health savings account.

Maya, 49, is a busy single mom and marketing executive. She was exhausted and overwhelmed by perimenopause. "I thought I needed to overhaul my whole life," she said. "But what I really needed was to stop trying to do everything." She started with ten minutes of morning movement. Within a month, she added a protein-rich breakfast and a nightly wind-down routine. "I gave myself a little bit of time each day, and the overwhelm eased. I started to feel like myself again."

"Progress, not punishment." These recovery habits are about finding gentle, practical ways to restore balance in your daily life.

Why Ten Minutes?

Because it's short enough to start and long enough to matter. Ten minutes lowers resistance. Psychologists call this the "minimum viable action." When the step feels small, your brain is more likely to say yes.

Neuroscience shows that even short bursts of activity can create new neural pathways (Doidge, 2007). And it just makes sense. You already have enough to juggle each day. Ten minutes feels doable. It breaks the all-or-nothing trap and keeps you consistent.

Ten minutes is also habit-forming. Every time you show up for yourself, even briefly, you prove you can be consistent. You build trust with yourself. Over time, those small wins add up to real progress. Think of it this way: ten minutes a day to change your next ten years.

Brain science tells us that small wins release dopamine, the "feel good" chemical, and help lower stress. Even short exercise sessions improve insulin sensitivity, stamina, and mood.

The research is clear too. In one study, adults aged 40–85 who added just ten minutes of moderate activity daily lowered their risk of death by 7%. With twenty extra minutes, the risk dropped by 13% (Zhao et al., 2019).

Each ten-minute session is a chance to listen to your body, care for yourself, and invest in your future. And your future self will thank you.

Tiny Habits for Big Change

Tiny is mighty.
BJ Fogg

Small shifts can create massive impact. Menopause offers a chance to pause and choose a new approach. You've spent years caring for others. Now it's time to care for yourself with compassion and wisdom. Healing doesn't come from hustling harder. It comes from replenishing yourself, one healthy meal, one glass of water, one moment of calm at a time.

When your body feels out of sync and your schedule is overloaded, the last thing you need is another long to do list. This is where tiny habits, small choices you can do in under a minute, make all the difference. Stanford behavior scientist BJ Fogg, creator of the Tiny Habits® method, explains that motivation comes and goes. But tiny actions tied to daily routines stick. The key is linking new habits to things you already do, like brushing your teeth or walking the dog.

Tracking habits can help too. A simple tracker with color-coded dots or checkmarks gives you visual proof of progress and keeps momentum going.

The Habit Loop

In *The Power of Habit*, Charles Duhigg explains that every habit follows the same loop.

Cue   **Craving**   **Response**   **Reward**

For example, walking into the kitchen in the morning might cue the desire for coffee. What you really crave isn't the coffee itself, it's the energy boost. The response is brewing the coffee. The reward is that first sip, which perks you up.

You can use this loop to build better habits. This method is called **habit stacking**.

"Before I [current habit], I will [new habit]."

For example:

- "Before I pour my morning coffee, I will drink a glass of water and take my vitamins."
- "After I finish the dinner dishes, I will go for a walk."

Pairing a new habit with an old one makes it easier to remember and more likely to stick.

Making Habits Stick

- To integrate a new habit successfully:

- Stack it with something you already do daily.

- Use clear cues that are easy to remember.

- Know your why and remind yourself why the habit matters.

- Reduce friction to make the habit simple to do.

- Make the reward satisfying to feel the relief, joy, or boost it brings.

When the reward feels good, your brain locks it in. That makes it easier to repeat tomorrow.

Start With the Why

Most people set goals around **outcomes** ("I want to lose weight") or **actions** ("I'll walk every day"). But the deepest and most lasting change comes from a shift in **identity**:

"I am someone who feels good in my body."

As Simon Sinek reminds us: start with why.

Why do you want to feel better? Who do you want to become?

You can become the kind of person who replenishes her energy by being more active on the weekend.

You can become the kind of person who shuts down email after 5 p.m. so evenings belong to family.

You can become the kind of person who packs a healthy lunch and takes time to sit outside and enjoy it.

The key is keeping your mind set on why you're making the change. That "why" is your motivation. It keeps you steady when life gets busy.

Over time, your perspective shifts. "I'm too busy to stop for lunch, I'll eat at my desk" becomes, "It would feel good to step outside and breathe fresh air."

Every time you follow through on a habit, you reinforce that identity. You're not just checking off a task, you're becoming the kind of person you want to be. Eventually, the habit is no longer a chore. It's simply part of who you are.

The Power of Compassionate Inquiry

How would your day look if you made choices based on what truly nurtures you?

When you let this question guide your daily decisions, you start to notice the small choices you make all day long. Some choices can drain you like poor diet, chronic stress, or lack of rest. Others can lift you up like nourishing food, gentle movement, or moments of calm. Over time, these choices add up and shape your well-being.

A blank journal can help you track these subtle changes. After a few days or weeks of writing, look back for patterns. Does your body keep asking for more rest, better hydration, or more movement? Do you notice symptoms such as racing thoughts, broken sleep, or sudden fatigue that you hadn't connected to menopause before?

These insights can guide you toward a daily rhythm that supports your needs, builds resilience, and honors this phase of life.

Keep track in your journal, and then use what you learn to adjust how you respond. It can make you wiser about your body. It helps you see what works, what doesn't, and how you can better care for yourself.

Self-care is never "done." It's an ongoing practice. Some days, you'll feel proactive and energetic. Other days, you'll simply do your best. Both count. Each small action you take to support your body, mind, and spirit adds up to a steadier, more resilient you.

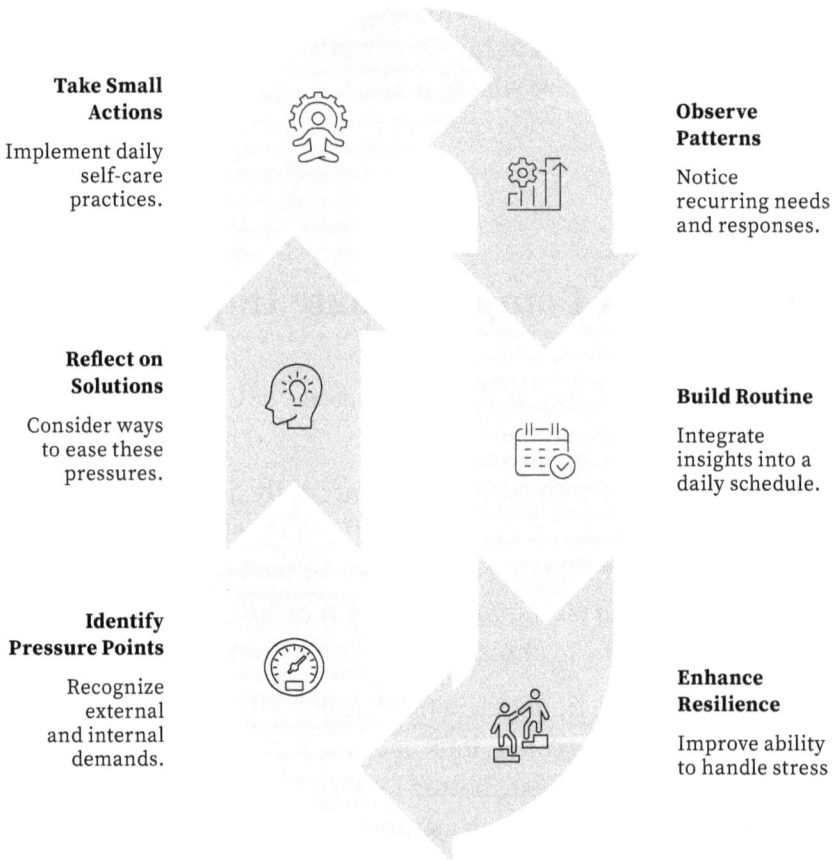

Take Small Actions

Implement daily self-care practices.

Observe Patterns

Notice recurring needs and responses.

Reflect on Solutions

Consider ways to ease these pressures.

Build Routine

Integrate insights into a daily schedule.

Identify Pressure Points

Recognize external and internal demands.

Enhance Resilience

Improve ability to handle stress

Do This Today

- Take ten minutes for something restorative.
- Walk around your neighborhood.
- Drink a glass of water with lemon.
- Eat a protein-rich snack.
- Take five deep breaths with your hands on your heart.
- Stretch your back.
- Sit in the sun with your eyes closed and listen to the world around you.

Reflection

Ask yourself: "What's one small thing I can do today that feels kind to my body?"

Listen closely. If you're tired, rest may be your kindness today. If you feel energetic, kindness might mean joyful movement such as dancing, yoga, pickleball, or swimming.

Chapter 2
Nourishment

---

*"Let food be thy medicine and
medicine be thy food."*

Hippocrates

In your twenties and thirties, you might have been able to pull off late-night pizza or skip meals without major consequences. You bounced back quickly or could keep going at full speed. But after you reach your forties, your body needs more deliberate care and high-quality nourishment to function well.

As we explored in Chapter 1, shifting estrogen levels change how your body responds to food. One key effect is less stable blood sugar, which can show up as energy crashes, irritability, or stronger cravings (Davis et al., 2015).

That's why your day-to-day food choices matter more than ever in midlife. Even small adjustments like balancing protein with carbs or limiting added sugar can help steady your energy and mood.

A healthy, balanced diet involves simple, mindful choices. A diet rich in whole foods helps establish a healthy gut biome, reduce inflammation, regulate hormones, and manage your weight. You can relieve many menopausal symptoms simply by focusing on an anti-inflammatory diet rich in whole foods. These symptoms include fatigue, hot flashes, brain fog, irritability, bloating, gas, constipation, breast tenderness, and joint pain.

This chapter takes a practical approach to adding healthier habits to your daily routine. The goal is to help you sustain healthy eating patterns that nourish your body, restore your sense of balance, and ultimately make you feel more vibrant and energetic.

Lena, 49, a busy project manager and mom of two, relied on cereal for breakfast, coffee midday, and pasta for dinner. She began waking up drenched in sweat. She felt out of sorts at night and crashed mid-morning at work. Her doctor ruled out thyroid issues, but her nutritionist spotted a pattern: blood sugar roller coasters and minimal protein. Lena started her day with a protein-rich breakfast and swapped white carbs for veggies and lentils. It helped her reclaim energy, curb hot flashes, and even sleep better.

Prioritize Protein

Blood sugar stability is key to hormone harmony. When you eat refined carbs or skip meals, your blood sugar spikes and then crashes. This forces your adrenal glands to pump out cortisol. Over time, this pattern contributes to insulin resistance, weight gain, fatigue, and mood swings (Kelley et al., 2002). The ups and downs strain your adrenal glands and leave you feeling depleted.

"After menopause, women need even more protein to maintain muscle mass, support mood, and boost metabolism," says Dr. Gabrielle Lyon, a functional medicine physician. Protein stabilizes blood sugar, supports muscle maintenance, and keeps you feeling fuller for longer. Studies show that protein-rich meals slow down digestion, reduce post-meal glucose spikes, and keep your energy levels steady throughout the day (Leidy et al., 2015). As a result, you can feel calmer, more balanced, and more resilient when you eat nutrient-dense meals.

As a general guide, include at least 20–30 grams of protein in each meal. Pair it with fiber-rich veggies and healthy fats like avocado, nuts, or olive oil. That could look like:

- Omelette with spinach and feta, plus a side of berries.
- Eggs with sautéed greens and avocado.
- Greek yogurt with chia seeds and berries.
- Lentil soup with a side of veggie-filled quinoa.
- Salad with avocado and grilled chicken.
- A handful of almonds with a boiled egg.
- Low-fat cheese and turkey lettuce wrap, with fresh fruit.

Sugar rushes are cheap. Stable energy is priceless. These combinations stabilize blood sugar, improve satiety, and help regulate key hormones like insulin and cortisol. Try to avoid eating just carbs on their own (like crackers or fruit). Whenever possible, pair carbs with protein. Also, eat smaller meals throughout the day if you notice your energy tends to crash.

Anti-Inflammatory Foods

Chronic inflammation can cause a host of problems: joint pain, poor digestion, fatigue, anxiety, depression, and brain fog. If you regularly consume processed foods, trans fats, sugary snacks, or alcohol, you might be dealing with chronic inflammation without even knowing it. Switching to an anti-inflammatory diet can bring considerable relief. Anti-inflammatory foods help heal your digestive system, support your immune system, balance hormones, and protect brain health.

Examples of anti-inflammatory foods include:

- Leafy greens (lettuce, spinach, kale, arugula).
- Berries (blueberries, strawberries, raspberries).
- Omega-3 fatty acid sources (salmon, walnuts, flaxseeds).
- Whole grains (brown rice, quinoa, buckwheat).
- Spices like turmeric and ginger (powerful anti-inflammatories).
- Green tea (loaded with antioxidants).

These foods help reduce oxidative stress, which can spike during hormonal changes (Zhao et al., 2019). As Dr. Mark Hyman writes in *The Pegan Diet* (2021), "Food isn't just calories. It's information. It talks to your DNA and tells it what to do." Your metabolism isn't broken, it's just waiting for new instructions. Anti-inflammatory foods provide strategic nourishment to your entire body, including your digestive, immune, nervous, and endocrine systems.

Gut-Brain Hormone Connection

Your gut microbiome affects how your body metabolizes estrogen, your immune function, and even your mental health. About 90% of the body's serotonin, the neurotransmitter that contributes to your sense of well-being, is made in your gut (Yano et al., 2015). Your gut microbiome influences everything from mood and metabolism to inflammation and hormone detoxification. If your digestion is sluggish or you feel bloated, chances are your hormones are also out of sync. If your digestion is off, everything else can feel off too. Bloating, brain fog, fatigue, and mood swings can all be symptoms of gut imbalance.

An anti-inflammatory, whole-food diet supports gut health. In addition to eating whole foods, try to incorporate:

- Fermented foods like yogurt, kefir, kimchi, or sauerkraut.
- Plenty of fiber from foods like black beans, brown rice, and sweet potatoes.
- Prebiotic sources like onions, garlic, and oats.

These additions create as much good bacteria in your gut as possible. Research shows that women with more diverse gut microbiota experience fewer menopause-related symptoms (Szeliga et al., 2021). This suggests that probiotics, prebiotics, and fiber can make a difference. It's also important for gut health to drink plenty of water. Whenever possible, avoid unnecessary antibiotics, excessive alcohol, ultra-processed foods, and stress. These can destroy the balance of good bacteria in your digestive system.

Soothe Joints Through Nutrition

Menopausal hormone changes can also make your joints ache. As estrogen levels decline, its anti-inflammatory protection diminishes. This leads to higher inflammation, which contributes to joint pain and stiffness. By choosing foods that fight inflammation (and cutting back on those that fuel it), you give your body the tools to calm achy knees, fingers, and hips.

Fill your plate with anti-inflammatory nutrition. An anti-inflammatory diet can act like natural medicine for your joints. Omega-3 fatty acids help reduce inflammatory chemicals in the body, easing joint pain. You can find these fats in fatty fish (such as salmon and sardines), as well as in flaxseeds, chia seeds, and walnuts. Brightly colored fruits and leafy green vegetables are packed with antioxidants and polyphenols that combat inflammation. Think of berries, spinach, kale, and broccoli for a vibrant, joint-friendly boost. Turmeric and ginger contain powerful compounds (like curcumin) that reduce inflammation and joint pain. You can enjoy these spices in a cup of ginger tea or in a mug of golden milk (made with turmeric).

Water keeps the cartilage in your joints well lubricated, which can reduce pain and that grinding sensation. Aim to drink water regularly throughout the day and include water-rich foods (soups, cucumbers, melons). Your joints are coated in synovial fluid, and it needs adequate hydration to do its job. On the flip side, try to moderate things that dry you out or ramp up inflammation. For example, too much alcohol or caffeine can dehydrate you and even trigger more inflammation. Enjoy that glass of wine or coffee in moderation. Similarly, easing up on sugary treats and refined carbs can pay off in less joint inflammation. Many women find that when they cut back on sugar and processed foods, their joint aches improve.

Your gut health and joint health are connected. The collection of microbes in your gut influences inflammation levels throughout your body. An imbalance in gut bacteria can increase systemic inflammation, which may aggravate joint pain. Scientific research shows that eating a diet rich in whole food and high in fiber will feed the good bacteria in your gut and help to lower inflammation. Fermented foods like yogurt, kefir, or sauerkraut introduce beneficial probiotics, while fiber from fruits, veggies, and whole grains acts as a prebiotic to nourish a healthy microbiome. Women with more diverse gut bacteria tend to have fewer menopause symptoms (aches and pains included). Caring for your gut with whole foods, fiber, and fermented foods, while limiting gut irritants like processed foods, sugar, and alcohol improves joint health too.

Food is a powerful ally during menopause. Every anti-inflammatory meal or snack helps your body heal. Over time, these small choices add up to joints that feel more comfortable. It might start with something as simple as adding ground flaxseed to your morning smoothie. Or choose a salad with olive oil dressing (rich in omega-3 and monounsaturated fats) for lunch. Bit by bit, you'll cushion your joints against the inflammation that comes with declining estrogen.

Find a Balanced Approach that Works for You

Pay attention to your biorhythms. Eating too close to bedtime, particularly heavy or sugar-laden meals, can interfere with melatonin production and disrupt sleep. To stay in harmony with your natural circadian rhythm, try to eat your last meal at least three hours before bedtime. Studies suggest finishing dinner by early evening and avoiding late-night snacks can improve metabolism and hormonal balance. Intermittent fasting (for example, not eating between 6 p.m. and 9 a.m.) can help with weight management and blood sugar control.

Embrace an anti-inflammatory whole foods diet. Build meals around colorful vegetables, fruits, whole grains, legumes, nuts, and seeds. These plant-based foods provide fiber, antioxidants, and phytonutrients that combat menopause-related inflammation and oxidative stress. Eating a "rainbow" of produce also gives you vitamins and minerals that support energy and hormone balance. Aim for healthy fats like olive oil and avocados as well.

Prioritize healthy fats. Include fatty fish (salmon, sardines, mackerel) or plant sources of omega-3s (ground flaxseed, chia seeds, walnuts) at least 2–3 times a week. These foods help reduce inflammation and support brain and heart health. Omega-3 fats balance hormones and may ease joint pain. Add a tablespoon of ground flax or chia to oatmeal or smoothies and snack on walnuts. Use olive oil or avocado oil for cooking and salad dressings (they're rich in anti-inflammatory monounsaturated fats).

Boost fiber intake for gut health. Eat plenty of fiber-rich foods like beans, lentils, oats, whole grains, fruits, and vegetables. Fiber feeds beneficial gut bacteria. High fiber diets are linked to steadier energy and improved insulin sensitivity (which often worsens after menopause). Aim for 25–35 grams of fiber each day from whole foods. For example, add berries to yogurt, include a side of legumes, or a whole grain like quinoa with your meals.

Integrate fermented and probiotic foods. Support your gut microbiome by eating fermented foods like yogurt, kefir, sauerkraut, kimchi, or kombucha. A healthy microbiome helps process estrogens and may improve mood, digestion, and even sleep. For example, have a serving of plain yogurt or kefir with berries at breakfast (fermented dairy provides probiotics and calcium). Fermented vegetables such as sauerkraut and pickles also add flavor and beneficial enzymes.

Eat phytoestrogen-rich whole foods. Incorporate foods with natural plant estrogens (isoflavones and lignans) such as soybeans (edamame, tofu), chickpeas, flaxseed, sesame seeds, and berries. Phytoestrogens may support bone health and cardiovascular health during menopause. For example, sprinkle ground flaxseed on cereal, or add tofu or tempeh to stir-fries and salads.

Focus on quality protein. To counter muscle and bone loss, include a good source of protein at every meal. Choose lean meats, fish, eggs, dairy, or plant proteins (beans, lentils, tofu, tempeh).

Balance meals for steady energy. Menopause lowers estrogen-driven insulin sensitivity, so balance carbohydrates with protein and fat to avoid energy crashes. Pair whole grains (brown rice, oats, quinoa) with protein and vegetables at meals. For example, make a stir-fry with brown rice, chicken or beans, and plenty of veggies. Avoid high-glycemic sugars and refined carbs that spike blood sugar. Keeping blood sugar stable can reduce fatigue, cravings, and mood swings. If you have pasta or bread, fill half your plate with vegetables or salad to balance the carbs.

Stay hydrated and be mindful of stimulants. Drink plenty of water throughout the day and include hydrating options like soups, herbal teas, and water-rich vegetables. Adequate fluids aid digestion, energy, and temperature regulation. Limit alcohol and caffeine (especially after mid-afternoon), as they can worsen hot flashes and disrupt sleep. Golden milk (made with turmeric, cinnamon, and ginger) can be a soothing bedtime ritual.

Inspiration for Whole Food Meals

Breakfast

- Omelette with spinach and feta, plus a side of berries.
- Greek yogurt bowl with chia seeds, walnuts, blueberries, and a drizzle of honey.
- Chickpea and veggie hash with turmeric and cumin, topped with a poached egg.
- Smoothie with unsweetened almond milk, frozen spinach, banana, plant protein, and flaxseeds.
- Overnight oats made with oats, almond milk, cinnamon, chia seeds, and topped with pumpkin seeds and berries.

Lunch

- Lentil salad with avocado and grilled chicken.
- Quinoa bowl with roasted sweet potatoes, kale, black beans, and tahini dressing.
- Turkey and hummus wrap in a whole grain wrap with mixed greens.
- Zucchini noodles with grilled shrimp, cherry tomatoes, and pesto.
- Stuffed bell peppers with ground turkey or lentils, brown rice, and herbs.

Snack

- A handful of almonds with a boiled egg.
- Apple slices with almond butter.
- Veggie sticks with hummus or guacamole.
- A square of dark chocolate with a few walnuts.

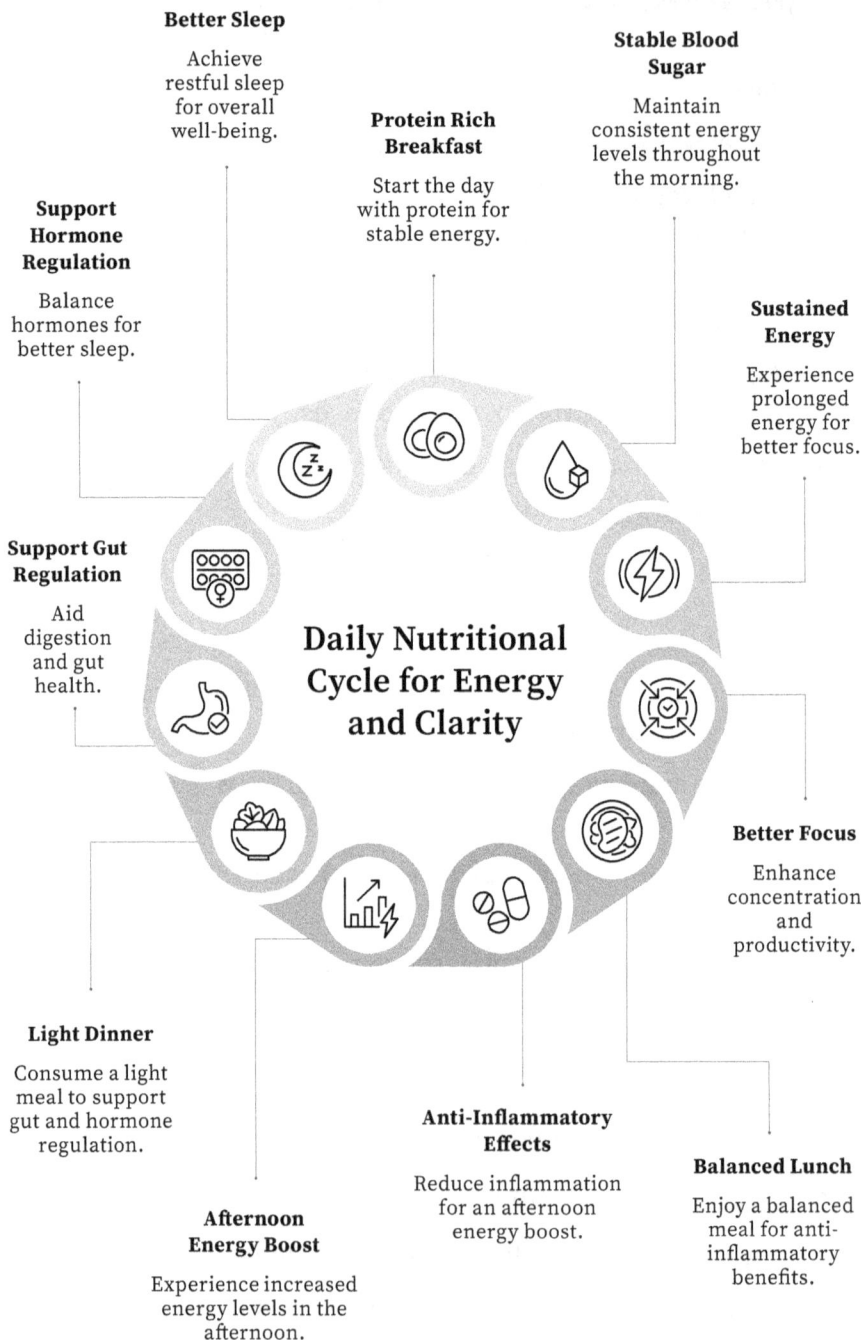

Daily Nutritional Cycle for Energy and Clarity

Better Sleep

Achieve restful sleep for overall well-being.

Protein Rich Breakfast

Start the day with protein for stable energy.

Stable Blood Sugar

Maintain consistent energy levels throughout the morning.

Support Hormone Regulation

Balance hormones for better sleep.

Sustained Energy

Experience prolonged energy for better focus.

Support Gut Regulation

Aid digestion and gut health.

Better Focus

Enhance concentration and productivity.

Light Dinner

Consume a light meal to support gut and hormone regulation.

Anti-Inflammatory Effects

Reduce inflammation for an afternoon energy boost.

Balanced Lunch

Enjoy a balanced meal for anti-inflammatory benefits.

Afternoon Energy Boost

Experience increased energy levels in the afternoon.

Nourishment as an Act of Self-Love

Menopause is not a shutdown. It's a power up. Healthy eating habits can revolutionize how you feel, and you can start to notice the difference right away. With a few smart nutrition changes, you can transform how you take care of your body's changing needs. Every colorful plate, every glass of water, every balanced snack is a small act of kindness toward yourself.

Kristin, 48, was a professor and a single mom who was used to being active, eating healthy, and going nonstop. But she started to realize that she was deeply exhausted all the time and often felt off her game. She woke with racing thoughts, experienced crashing fatigue, and suddenly had a lot of new aches and pains. She switched to a whole foods diet with fermented foods and probiotics, and she changed her evening wind down routine to include restorative yoga and reading before bedtime instead of television. Once or twice a week, she integrated a 5-minute cold plunge. Within a few weeks, the racing thoughts, crashing fatigue, and achiness disappeared.

"I resisted the diet change at first, because I thought I was a healthy eater. But once I realized how depleted I felt, I changed. Gut health doesn't happen overnight, but when you heal your gut with whole foods, the difference is profound. The cold plunge is surprisingly effective: it helps with inflammation, and it also triggers a sense of euphoria that I've started to look forward to each week. I feel more embodied and centered when I give myself the time I need to take care of myself."

Do This Today

Integrate smart prep sessions into your weekly meal planning. For instance:

- Make a batch of hard-boiled eggs for quick protein.
- Chop veggies and store them in glass containers for easy salads or stir fries.
- Prep nutrient dense snacks like nuts, fruit, dark chocolate, hummus, or low-fat cheese.
- Set up simple breakfasts, like overnight oats or smoothie packs (greens, fruit, protein powder, seeds).
- Freeze pre-cooked brown rice or quinoa in single portions for quick, high fiber meals.

Reflection

Ask yourself: "When during the week do I usually struggle most with healthy eating? How could ten minutes of prep make that moment easier?"

Chapter 3
Better Sleep, Better Days

———

"Good sleep is not a luxury. It's a non-negotiable foundation of hormonal balance, mental clarity, and emotional resilience."

Dr. Shelby Harris, clinical psychologist and sleep specialist

———

Feeling tired isn't a character flaw. It's a hormone call for help. For many women in midlife, sleep becomes difficult. Fluctuating hormones can interfere with both the quality and quantity of rest. Fortunately, there are science-backed tools to support both the prevention and recovery from poor sleep. If you suffer from night sweats, racing thoughts, or disrupted sleep, you can start to integrate some simple, evidence-based habits to improve your sleep. These changes can address menopausal symptoms, enhance your sleep hygiene, and train your brain to relax into a new nighttime rhythm that works for you.

The Power of Routine

You can't be the healthiest version of yourself
if you're chronically sleep-deprived.
Sleep isn't selfish it's essential.
Dr. Sara Gottfried, The Hormone Cure

Regulating your circadian rhythm throughout the day leads to better sleep at night. This means even your morning and daytime habits affect your nighttime rest. For instance, start your morning with sunlight. Open the curtains to let natural light in, or step outside to help your body wake up. During the day, get some exercise early. Also, stop drinking caffeine by early afternoon so it has time to leave your system before bedtime. In the evening, avoid overstimulation and keep the lights low to cue your body for sleep.

You can greatly improve the quality of your rest by establishing a calm nightly wind-down routine and sleeping in a cool, dark, quiet space. Your bedroom should be a sleep sanctuary. The right environment can make a world of difference. A quiet, cooler room helps your body relax. According to experts, your room should be cool, dark, quiet, and clutter-free. Temperature plays a big role. Aim for around 65–68°F (18–20°C). Cooler body temperatures trigger sleep, helping you fall asleep faster and stay asleep longer. Try using a fan, blackout curtains, and a white noise machine.

Sleep scientist Matthew Walker says that when it comes to good sleep, "Regularity is king." A consistent sleep schedule helps you establish a rhythm that benefits your sleep over time. Following a regular wind-down routine signals to your mind and body that it's time to slow down and rest. Arianna Huffington, in her book The Sleep Revolution, calls her own bedtime ritual "sacrosanct," emphasizing how vital it is to separate the day from the night. She takes an Epsom salt bath and prolongs it when feeling anxious to truly decompress. Interestingly, a warm shower or bath before bed increases blood flow to your skin and leads to a drop in core body temperature when you get out. That cooling can enhance deep sleep by up to 15% (Haghayegh et al., 2019).

Start your wind-down routine about an hour before bed. This gives your body time to transition toward sleep. Your routine might include sipping herbal tea, meditating, journaling, reading, or spending quiet time with loved ones. Dim the lights and turn off electronic devices to prepare your brain for sleep.

Understanding Your Sleep Window

Your body has a built-in sleep rhythm, a personal "sleep window" that opens each night when your brain and body are most ready to drift off. This sweet spot is when melatonin naturally rises and your urge to rest is at its peak. Falling asleep during this time helps your brain develop a healthy sleep habit. Over time, it can dramatically improve the quality of your rest.

If you miss that window (for example, if you stay up scrolling on your phone or watching one more episode), your alertness can bounce back just as you're trying to wind down. Suddenly, you feel wide awake, even though you were yawning an hour ago. That's your circadian rhythm getting confused, and it can lead to fragmented or restless sleep. As you wind down each night, get in the habit of noticing when you are approaching your sleep window.

If you regularly struggle to fall asleep, try gradually resetting your bedtime. Move it earlier by 15–30 minutes every few nights until you feel naturally sleepy during your ideal window again.

Skip the binge-watching or last-minute chores if they're nudging your bedtime later. Honoring your sleep window can make falling asleep (and staying asleep) much easier.

You can also experiment during quieter weeks or weekends. Notice when you start to feel naturally drowsy, and track how long you sleep when left undisturbed. Tools like sleep diaries or wearable trackers can help. Once you spot your window, set a gentle reminder to start winding down when that time is near.

When Sleep Just Doesn't Happen

Even with the best routine, there are nights when sleep doesn't come easily. Hormonal shifts during menopause can make it harder to fall asleep, stay asleep, or feel rested in the morning. If you wake up in the middle of the night, don't panic. There are strategies to manage sleep interruptions without spiraling into insomnia.

#1: Calm Anxiety

The worry spiral of "What if I can't sleep tonight?" will raise stress hormones and make sleep even harder. Instead, remind yourself that this is temporary and not dangerous. Focus on relaxing, not "trying" to sleep. Do a few rounds of slow breathing or try progressive muscle relaxation (tensing and releasing each muscle group one by one). You can also use guided meditations, yoga nidra, or soft background noise (like brown noise or pink noise) to calm a racing mind. Another technique is the "mental stroll": visualize yourself in detail, walking through a familiar, soothing place. This kind of visualization distracts your mind from worry and can lull you back to sleep.

#2: Get Out of Bed

If you can't fall back asleep within twenty minutes, get up and do something relaxing. For example, read a book or sip a cup of herbal "bedtime" tea (like chamomile, lavender, passionflower, valerian, or licorice root). Keep the lights low and avoid screens. Return to bed only when you feel truly sleepy again.

#3: Cool Down

If a hot flash or night sweat jolts you awake, try to cool off. Splash cool water on your face, sip cold water, or flip your pillow to the cool side. An ice pack under your neck can help too. If you often wake up hot, consider moisture-wicking pajamas and breathable sheets.

#4: Ease Discomfort

For restless legs or nighttime cramps, use a warm heating pad or take a magnesium-rich Epsom salt bath before bed. Gentle leg stretches can also relieve nighttime tension and twitching.

#5: Resist Oversleeping

It's tempting to sleep in or take long naps after a poor night's sleep, but that can throw off your rhythm. Try to wake up at your usual time. If you're truly exhausted, take a short 20-minute power nap in the early afternoon rather than a long nap. Keeping a steady wake time will reset your sleep drive for the next night.

#6: Handle Early Wake-ups

Waking at 4 a.m. and feeling wide awake can be frustrating. Try to stay calm and relaxed. Practice deep breathing or listen to calming sounds to help lull you back to sleep. If you remain wide awake after a while, follow the routine above: get up, do something quiet, then return to bed when you feel sleepy. Avoid ruminating or doom scrolling on your phone, stress will only make you feel more tired later.

#7: Try Gentle Sleep Aids

If you feel anxious and can't unwind, consider a small dose of melatonin or magnesium glycinate an hour or two before bed. Even simple aids like a few drops of lavender oil on your pillow can help ease you into sleep. (Always talk to your doctor about using supplements, especially if you take other medications.)

Lori, a 49-year-old woman navigating the ups and downs of menopause, found herself lying awake each night, feeling restless and drained. She had tried everything—medications, a better mattress, and even supplements—but sleep continued to elude her. Frustrated, she sought advice and began to prioritize a calming bedtime routine.

Lori started by dimming the lights an hour before bed and sipping a cup of chamomile tea. After that, she would stretch or do a few rounds of deep breathing exercises. Soon, she found that the simple act of winding down signaled her body that it was time for rest. Making sleep a ritual gave her the space to relax and let go of the day's stresses.

Natural Sleep Support

You can experiment with natural ways to support your evening routine for better sleep. Here are some practical, proven sleep allies that help your brain feel safe enough to drift off and stay asleep. Pick one, or a few, and make them part of your routine:

Eye Masks

Block out stray light that can suppress melatonin (a hormone often reduced during menopause). Complete darkness helps reset your natural sleep chemistry.

Weighted Blankets

The light, even pressure can calm your nervous system, lower anxiety, and promote deeper sleep.

Nasal Strips

These open up your nasal passages and reduce mouth breathing, snoring, and dry mouth.

Visualization

Guided imagery exercises can soothe cortisol-fueled insomnia. For example, mentally walk through a place where you feel at peace, and let the vivid details relax your mind.

Low Light

Keep your bedroom lighting dim in the evening. Low light helps your body produce melatonin and prepares you for sleep.

Herbal Teas

Varieties like chamomile, valerian, and passionflower have gentle, calming effects. These herbs may ease anxiety and support relaxation by acting on GABA receptors in the brain, similar to how anti-anxiety medications work (Srivastava et al., 2010).

Magnesium

This mineral (especially magnesium glycinate or citrate) is widely used to help with sleep. Research shows magnesium can improve sleep quality and reduce early morning awakening in older adults (Abbasi et al., 2012). It may also ease muscle cramps that disturb sleep.

L-theanine

An amino acid found in green tea, L-theanine promotes relaxation without causing drowsiness. It boosts GABA and serotonin, neurotransmitters that calm the nervous system. In one study, L-theanine supplementation improved sleep in adults

(Bulman, 2025). This is often recommended for anxious perimenopausal women.

Valerian Root and Fennel

These have shown promise for menopause-related sleep issues. Clinical trials suggest valerian can reduce the time it takes to fall asleep and improve sleep quality in menopausal women (Taavoni et al., 2020). Fennel has been linked to fewer hot flashes and less sleep disruption (Farshbaf Khalili et al., 2020).

Melatonin

In low doses (0.3–1 mg), melatonin can help regulate sleep timing and improve sleep quality in postmenopausal women. One study found that prolonged-release melatonin improved sleep and reduced vasomotor symptoms in postmenopausal participants (Lemoine et al, 2011). Use it sparingly, so you don't build up a tolerance or dependency.

Do This Today

Refine your wind-down routine.

- Set a calming alarm one hour before bed as a reminder to start slowing down.

- Dim the lights and unplug from screens.

- Choose a few calming rituals: have a warm cup of golden milk or herbal tea, read a book, write in a journal, do some restorative yoga stretches, or give yourself a gentle foot or neck massage.

- Notice when your sleep window opens (when you start feeling drowsy). Use that moment as your cue to get into bed.

Use the following sleep hygiene diary to help you find your ideal sleep patterns.

Reflection

Ask yourself: "What small shift in my evening routine makes the biggest difference in how I feel the next morning?" Use this insight as you track your habits in the Sleep Hygiene Diary.

Sleep Hygiene Diary

Use this simple diary to track your natural sleep window and evening routine habits for one week. Check in with yourself each night and note any patterns. This will help you fine-tune your bedtime routine and improve sleep quality.

Day	Sleep Window Time	Lights-Off Time	Estimated Sleep Time	Wake-Up Time	Notes: Mood, hot flashes, disruptions?
Monday					
Tuesday					
Wednesday					
Thursday					
Friday					
Saturday					
Sunday					

A printable version is available at
https://menopause.habitkind.store/bonus
(or simply scan the QR code)

SCAN ME

Chapter 4
Mental Well-Being

———

"Menopause is a second puberty. Your body is changing again, and it deserves the same care, curiosity, and compassion."

Dr. Jen Gunter

———

If you are feeling irritable, scattered, and exhausted, you are not alone. These feelings are common during the menopause transition when your hormonal balance shifts. Menopause symptoms can affect your brain, your emotions, and your mental clarity. It's time we talked about it.

Dr. Louann Brizendine, neuropsychiatrist and author of *The Female Brain*, explains that estrogen acts like a master regulator of many brain functions. Its decline can feel like "a dimmer switch being turned down." And it's not all in your head; it's in your hormones.

Estrogen plays a role in modulating neurotransmitters like serotonin, dopamine, and norepinephrine, chemicals that regulate mood, focus, and memory. When estrogen declines, the brain's chemistry shifts, leading to brain fog, mood swings, and sleep disruption. During this time, it helps to become aware of your mental state as it fluctuates throughout the day.

Practice mindful awareness by noticing how efficiently you are processing information, how you feel, and what your state of mind is. With this awareness, you can begin to use interventions that help bring you back to an optimal state of mind.

If you are having trouble finding words, difficulty concentrating, or experiencing irritability, anxiety, or emotional sensitivity, you are not alone. These symptoms are common. When you recognize the symptoms, try to name it. "This is hormonal." Then, try hydrating, grounding yourself with some deep breathing, and take a short walk or stretch break to increase your circulation and refocus your attention. Give yourself five minutes to rest and reset, then come back to what you were doing.

Circuit Breakers Interrupt the Loop

When you're overwhelmed, foggy, snappy, or exhausted, it's often because you're doing too much too fast. In these moments, it can help to break the rhythm. That's where "circuit breakers" come in. Just as a fuse flips when an electrical system is overloaded, your mind and body need ways to interrupt the flow of stress, stimulation, and scattered energy. These "circuit breakers" are strategic resets that protect your mental bandwidth and restore clarity, calm, and control.

They are especially important in menopause because your cognitive load often increases, and you don't recover from stress as easily as you did when you were younger. If you pay attention to your symptoms, they can teach you what your body needs in order to function better. For example, brain fog can be a sign that you need to conserve energy. Mood swings might indicate that your cortisol levels are high. By using circuit breakers, consciously pausing and redirecting your effort, you can function better and not hit a breaking point.

Think of your mental energy as a limited resource. You can only do so much before you start to lose effectiveness. Not everything that demands your time deserves your energy. Decision fatigue and overcommitment spike cortisol. Can you get in the habit of cutting out non-essential tasks to make space for recovery?

You also need more space to think, rest, and recharge. Can you build in buffer zones between meetings or errands to give yourself breathing room? In addition to buffer zones, make time for silence. Quiet time counteracts sensory overload, overstimulation, and racing thoughts. Also, simplifying your environment (a bit of minimalism) can soothe mental fatigue and anxiety. Create surroundings that calm your mind by reducing clutter.

If you tend to be a people-pleaser, use circuit breakers to interrupt the urge to say "yes" to everything. Establish a personal

48-hour rule before committing to new responsibilities, so you have time to think it over. You could also use a "soft no," for example, "I can't this month, but maybe later." Give yourself permission to cancel non-essential plans if you are feeling depleted and need to restore your energy.

To reduce cognitive overload, prioritize essential tasks. Remind yourself that "not everything that matters, matters right now." Practice batching similar tasks to reduce constant switching. For instance, do meal planning or outfit planning for the week all at once. Simplify decisions whenever possible. Put routine healthy choices on autopilot so they require less thought. Automatic habits can make healthy choices frictionless, because you're not overthinking them.

You don't shrink during menopause. You sharpen. Your aim is to take care of your mental and emotional well-being by noticing when you're starting to burn out or spiral, before it happens. Recognize the early signs of mental or emotional fatigue and take action to interrupt the cycle so you can rest and recharge. Your well-being requires this kind of attention and care, and there are many strategies to build resilience into your daily routine.

Michelle, 49, was always the high energy one. The plate spinner. She felt like she was the "I've got this" woman. Until she didn't.

"I thought I was just burnt out. I was drained, resentful, and short fused. I chalked it up to stress deadlines, parenting, life. But the truth? I was experiencing both burnout and menopause."

Her symptoms overlapped: fatigue, brain fog, mood swings. It took years for her to connect the dots. When she finally did, everything changed. She stopped pushing herself to the point of crashing. She built in regular recovery time.

"I started checking in with my energy like I check my phone battery often, and without guilt."

Strategies to Support Focus

Expressive Writing

Give your brain a daily cleanse by writing out your thoughts. Spend 3–5 minutes writing down everything that is worrying you or taking up mental space. Be honest about what's bothering you. (Feel free to tear up the paper afterward.)

Gratitude Journaling

Write down 3–5 things you're thankful for right now. Focusing on positive things triggers dopamine and serotonin. In fact, research shows that a gratitude practice can lower cortisol by about 23%, leading to a calmer outlook (Khorrami, 2020). Even on tough days, noting a few things you're grateful for can shift your thinking patterns and reframe your mindset.

Micro-Doses of Exercise

Neuroscientist Wendy Suzuki emphasizes the mood-boosting power of short bursts of movement. Do sixty seconds of jumping jacks, dancing, squats, or any quick exercise. Even brief movement can raise endorphins and clear your mind.

Hydrate

Take water breaks. Often, what feels like brain fog or fatigue is actually mild dehydration. Drinking water can refresh your mind.

Speed Breathing

Do a short burst of faster breathing (without hyperventilating) to boost alertness. This can raise norepinephrine in the brain and help wake you up.

Long-Distance Focus

Look away from your screen and focus on a distant object for a minute. Staring at something far away forces your brain to adjust focus, which can sharpen your attention and relieve eye strain. It also gives your mind a quick reset from intense close-up work.

Breathwork to Reduce Stress

Belly Breathing

Inhale slowly through your nose, letting your belly (not your chest) rise. Then exhale gently. This diaphragmatic breathing stimulates your vagus nerve and activates the parasympathetic "rest and digest" system. Just a few minutes of belly breathing can slow your heart rate, ease anxiety, and raise serotonin while lowering stress hormones.

Box Breathing

Inhale through your nose for a count of four. Hold your breath for a count of four. Exhale for a count of four and then hold again for four. This "four-square" breathing pattern boosts GABA (a calming brain chemical) and quiets racing thoughts. Box breathing is a simple way to reduce anxiety in the moment.

Alternate Nostril Breathing

Close your right nostril and inhale slowly through your left nostril. Then close your left nostril and exhale through the right. Inhale through the right nostril, then switch to exhale out of the left. Continue alternating sides with each breath. This yogic technique balances your nervous system. Just a few minutes of alternate nostril breathing can lower stress and help you feel centered.

Resonant Breathing

Breathe in for 5 seconds and out for 5 seconds (around 6 breaths per minute). This slow, even breathing pattern can sharpen focus and give you a mild dopamine boost to counteract brain fog. It's also inherently calming and can be done anywhere.

Movement and Stretching

Brisk 10-Minute Walk or Dance

A quick burst of aerobic movement can raise endorphins and serotonin (natural mood lifters) while lowering stress hormones. Take a fast 10-minute walk or dance to a favorite song. The increased blood flow and muscle movement will release tension and give you a little mood boost.

Stretch Break

Spend 5–10 minutes doing simple stretches or yoga poses. For example, reach your arms overhead, then fold forward to touch your toes. Try a warrior pose (one foot forward in a lunge, back leg straight, arms extended) and then a reverse warrior pose (from the lunge, reach one arm up and back while resting your other hand on your back leg). These poses open up tight hips and stretch your spine, helping you feel grounded. Just a few calming yoga poses can lower cortisol. Holding a stretch while breathing deeply increases circulation and releases built-up tension.

Shoulder Rolls and Neck Stretches

Shrug your shoulders up to your ears, then roll them back and down. Gently tilt your head side to side to stretch your neck. We often carry stress in our neck and shoulders. By releasing these muscles, you send signals to your brain that it's okay to relax. This can reduce the feeling of being "on edge." Regularly doing these stretches helps break the cycle of tension.

Somatic Nervous System Resets

Progressive Muscle Relaxation (5–10 Minutes)

Tense each major muscle group in your body for a few seconds, then let it go, working from your feet up to your head. For example, curl your toes and tense your feet, then release. Move to your calves, thighs, and so on. The contrast between tension and release helps cut down physical stress signals. Studies show this technique can reduce stress and cortisol levels by around 8–10% (Chellew et al., 2015). As your muscles relax, you'll feel anxiety decrease and a sense of calm set in.

Earlobe Massage (2–3 Minutes)

Gently rub and tug your earlobes and the area just behind your ears. This stimulates branches of the vagus nerve located there. Activating the vagus nerve through gentle ear massage has been shown to lower cortisol and boost serotonin. It's a simple self-soothing trick that can produce a calming effect and help shift your nervous system toward relaxation.

Self-Hug (2–3 Minutes)

Wrap your arms around yourself and squeeze gently, as if giving yourself a hug. This comforting pressure can trigger the release of oxytocin (the "cuddle hormone"). Even self-hugs or holding your own hand can reduce stress. Research shows that self-soothing touch lowers cortisol levels (Dreisoerner et al., 2021). When stress spikes, a self-hug can signal to your brain that you are safe and supported, helping you calm down.

Sensory Interventions

Laughter Break

Watch a funny video clip, recall a hilarious memory, or talk to someone who makes you laugh. Laughter floods your body with oxygen and triggers the release of endorphins and other feel-good neurochemicals. It also revs up your heart and muscles and then relaxes them. This cycle leaves you feeling lighter and calmer. Even a quick laugh can break the stress cycle and improve your mood.

Sound Therapy

Play an upbeat song to get a quick boost of energy and dopamine, or listen to soothing music or nature sounds to relax. Music can raise dopamine and serotonin, and lower cortisol. You can also sing or hum along. Humming (like chanting "om") creates vibrations that stimulate the vagus nerve, which helps you relax.

Light Therapy

Step outside into natural light for a few minutes. Sunlight prompts your brain to release serotonin, improving your mood and alertness. A short walk outdoors, especially in a green space, can significantly lower cortisol. If you're short on time, even standing by a window and looking at the sky for a minute can help reset your mind and reduce fogginess.

Grounding Exercise

Use your five senses to anchor yourself in the present. Look around and name five things you can see. Then four things you can feel (your feet on the floor, your clothing on your skin, etc.). Then three things you can hear right now. Two things you can smell. Finally, take one deep breath and think of one thing you're grateful for or know to be true. This "5-4-3-2-1" grounding technique pulls you out of anxious thoughts and back into the here and now.

Cold Therapy

Splash cold water on your face or press a cool washcloth against your forehead and cheeks. The sudden cold triggers a "dive reflex," which activates the parasympathetic nervous system. This slows your heart rate and calms you down. You'll often feel more clear-headed and relaxed after a quick cold splash or a cold pack on the back of your neck.

Each of these quick resets works by engaging your vagus nerve, balancing stress hormones, or releasing mood-supporting chemicals in your brain. Use them whenever you feel a sense of overwhelm, brain fog, or crankiness creeping in. These mini breaks remind your body that it's safe and remind your brain that it's capable. Best of all, each one takes ten minutes or less to help recharge your system.

For Linda, 48, menopause was a wake-up call.

"At first, I felt lost after sleepless nights, mood swings, and a fog that made me feel like a stranger in my own body. But instead of giving in to the chaos, I chose to listen. I chose to learn. And slowly, I reclaimed my energy, my power, and my peace. This chapter of life has become a doorway. Not an ending, but a beginning. I'm not who I used to be, and I'm proud of that."

"I now make healthy life choices with movement at the center. Movement became my medicine. I used to think workouts needed to be intense to 'count,' but menopause taught me otherwise. Now, I move because it feels good. I dance in the kitchen, stretch before bed, and take walks that clear my head. Moving reconnects me to my body, helps me manage my symptoms, and reminds me that strength is built one step at a time."

"Prioritizing fun and family changed everything. I stopped glorifying busyness. I started saying yes to game nights, beach walks, and spontaneous road trips. I let laughter back into my life. My

relationships grew stronger when I made space for joy, not just as a reward, but as a daily necessity. My family sees me differently now, not just as a provider or planner, but as a woman who lives with intention and makes room for what matters most."

"I feel great because I chose a different professional path. A few years ago, I made a bold choice. I stepped away from the hustle that once defined me, and into work that feels meaningful and aligns with my values. It wasn't easy, I'd spent years climbing a ladder that didn't lead where I wanted to go. But deep down, I knew I needed to change. Choosing a path that honors my energy, creativity, and well-being changed everything. I traded burnout for balance, and I haven't looked back."

"I feel happy when I reflect on my life today. There's a calm in my days now, a sense of joy that comes from within. It's not about perfection or having everything figured out, but about knowing that I show up for myself every day. I smile more. I sleep better. I move with purpose. I feel connected to who I am becoming, and that feeling is priceless."

Mood Swing Interventions

Somatic Release

Shake it out. Stand up and vigorously shake your arms, hands, and even your hips to dissipate excess cortisol or adrenaline. If you feel a surge of anger or frustration, channel it by shaking out that explosive energy in your body.

Stop The Story

When you catch yourself in a negative thought spiral, say "STOP" out loud. Interrupt the cycle. Remind yourself that you are not the anxious story your brain is spinning. This breaks the loop of stress-amplifying thoughts.

Speed Walk

Use movement to burn off a mood swing. A brisk walk can help release built-up emotional energy. As the saying goes, motion burns emotion. Let your leg muscles work through whatever is overwhelming your mind.

Do This Today

Practice a moment of radical honesty with yourself to avoid pushing too hard or ignoring your own needs. Remember, radical honesty can be kind and gentle. It's not about being harsh. Pause and acknowledge how you actually feel or what you truly need right now. By openly recognizing what your body or mind is asking for, you can set healthier boundaries, lighten your mental load, and protect your well-being.

Reflection

Ask yourself, "What is one small change I can make to reduce my mental load and conserve my energy?" Be honest about what you need to take care of yourself and give yourself permission to make that change.

Chapter 5
Muscle, Balance, and Movement

———

"Exercise is the closest thing we have to a magic pill. It changes your brain, your muscles, your metabolism, and even your mood."

Dr. Mark Hyman, *The UltraMind Solution*

———

This chapter looks at one of the unsung heroes during menopause: your muscles. Starting in your thirties, muscle mass naturally begins to decline. Muscle is important for many aspects of your health and well-being. It burns more calories than fat, even at rest, which is why having more muscle helps support your metabolism, weight, and energy. Muscle also protects your joints, regulates blood sugar, and even boosts mood by releasing hormones called myokines.

As estrogen wanes, it changes your muscle tissue, fat distribution, energy, and even how you bounce back from a bad night's sleep. Lower estrogen levels can lead to loss of muscle mass and a slower metabolism. When estrogen declines, inflammation rises, recovery slows, and your body becomes less efficient at maintaining lean tissue. It's a vicious cycle that can lead to unwanted weight gain. This cycle is even harder to break because women also experience a drop in testosterone in midlife. Lower testosterone is linked to reduced vitality and motivation (Bianchi et al., 2021; Gatenby & Simpson, 2024).

The good news is that you can rebuild muscle and boost metabolism. In one study, postmenopausal women who added resistance training to their routine increased their muscle strength, improved their body composition and bone density, and sped up their metabolism in just twelve weeks. Resistance training can involve lifting weights (dumbbells, medicine balls, kettlebells), using resistance bands, or even using your own body weight to strengthen your muscles. Challenging your muscles causes them to grow. Strength training also helps your body use insulin more efficiently, burn more calories, regulate metabolism, and maintain energy. Emerging research suggests that regular strength training can stimulate the release of IGF-1 (Insulin-like Growth Factor 1), a hormone tied to muscle growth, repair, and even brain health (Borst et al., 2001).

Karen, 52, never saw herself as someone who exercised. But she got fed up with feeling lethargic and out of shape. She chose a bodyweight strength training video on YouTube and followed along. To her surprise, it was fun. She loved the upbeat challenge and the boost of energy it gave her. Over time, she felt more confident as her endurance and core strength improved.

Stronger Muscles, Stronger Bones

Think of fitness as preparing you for your future self. The stronger your muscles, the stronger your bones. Resistance training can increase bone density and protect against osteoporosis. It also improves joint stability, which means a lower chance of falls and fractures.

To begin resistance training, start slow and gradually increase the weight and repetitions. Use enough resistance that your muscles feel challenged, but not so much that you lose good form. Muscles build when they are challenged progressively over time, with rest between sets and between workout sessions. If you consistently increase the challenge, after a few weeks you will start to feel the results. Seeing visible muscle definition may take longer, but be patient—it will come.

If you haven't been getting enough protein, or if you have chronic stress or haven't exercised much, you might feel weak when you start. Don't worry, muscle can be rebuilt at any age. Focus on three basic guidelines: be consistent, eat nutrient-dense meals with plenty of protein, and give yourself time to recover. Here's a bit more about each factor:

Be Consistent

Ten minutes of resistance training can make a measurable difference if you do it regularly. Start with bodyweight moves (like squats and wall push-ups) and build up. Count your repetitions to stay consistent. Perform a set of 8–12 reps, rest for about a minute, and repeat. As you get stronger, increase the challenge by adding weight or intensity.

Get Plenty of Protein

Your muscles are made of protein. During menopause, your body needs more protein to preserve lean muscle. The exact amount depends on your weight and activity level. As a general guideline, aim for 20–25 grams of protein per meal to fuel your body and keep blood sugar steady. (See Chapter 2: Nourishment for more on the importance of protein.)

Prioritize Recovery

Muscles grow while you rest, not while you lift. In addition to getting plenty of sleep, make sure you hydrate and eat magnesium-rich foods (like bananas, almonds, and leafy greens) to aid in muscle recovery.

Strength in Balance

Muscle is your midlife armor. Strengthening your core muscles (in your abdomen, back, hips, and pelvis) improves your posture, stability, and balance. Core strength protects against back pain, prevents falls, and makes everyday movements like standing, walking, squatting, lifting, and bending easier. Balance is part of your body's equilibrium (steadiness), which can be affected by menopause because estrogen influences your vestibular (balance) system. Good balance isn't only about your core. It's also about strengthening the muscles in your ankles, feet, and knees. Exercises that involve squatting, lifting, or balancing on one leg can improve your proprioception (your sense of your body's position in space) and dynamic stability.

Truths About Exercise After 40

- Cardio supports your heart, and strength training protects muscle and bone.
- It's never too late to build strength.
- Resistance training shapes lean, defined muscle.

- Just 10–15 minutes a day makes a difference.
- Balance strength, cardio, and recovery for best results.
- Exercise helps prevent both physical and cognitive decline.

10-Minute Strength Workouts

Ten minutes of resistance training is enough to begin stimulating muscle growth, but you have to do it regularly to see a difference. So treat your workouts like appointments, and show up for yourself. Don't train for your **summer** body—train for your **grandmother** body. If you don't see yourself as a "weightlifter," you might prefer the idea of functional fitness. **Functional fitness** focuses on movements that increase your strength and stability in daily activities, so you can move through your life with ease.

Functional fitness aims to stabilize your joints and strengthen your core for better mobility and stability, ultimately reducing your chance of fall-related injuries. Its goal is to help you move through your day with more independence and ease. Find the reason that motivates you to push yourself a little with each workout to maximize your muscle-building effort. Then start with some simple foundational resistance moves, like squats, wall push-ups, lunges, or crunches with a medicine ball. If you have joint concerns, try a chair workout with dumbbells or a resistance band.

Strength Circuit	Daily Circuit	Stability
Squats	Squats	Chair Pose
Wall Push-ups	Wall Push-ups	Chair pose on Tiptoes
Glute Bridges	Wide-legged Squat	Tree Pose
Modified Plank	Arm Circles (each direction)	Plié Squats
Lunges	Chair Pose (against wall)	Plié Squats on Tiptoes

Perform each move for 1-minute.

Repeat each circuit 2-3 times per week.

Movement is Medicine

So far we've focused on building muscle through strength training, a crucial piece of the puzzle. Equally important is how you move throughout the day. Movement isn't just formal exercise. It's every step you take, every stretch, every flight of stairs. All of these daily movements add up. In fact, research shows that even if you exercise regularly, sitting for too long during the rest of the day can still be harmful.

Breaking up long periods of sitting with short bursts of activity can lower your risk of heart disease and even death. One study found that women who reduced their sedentary time by just one hour per day cut their risk of heart disease by 26%. Those movement breaks did not have to be intense; even light activity helped ("Long Periods of Sedentary Behavior may Increase Cardiovascular Risk in Older Women," 2019).

Your body was built to move, not sit still.

The message is clear: all movement counts. Every time you walk during a phone call or take the stairs instead of the elevator, you're doing something positive for your health. These little "movement snacks" keep your metabolism active and your joints lubricated. In contrast, when you stay still, your muscles burn less sugar and your blood sugar can creep up. Long stretches of sitting also increase inflammation and stiffness in your body.

But if you get up and move for even a few minutes, you help regulate your blood sugar and blood pressure. You'll likely notice an energy and mood boost too. In one experiment, participants who took a 5-minute walking break every half hour had much lower blood sugar spikes and blood pressure. They also reported better mood and less fatigue by the end of the day ("Rx for Prolonged Sitting: A Five-Minute Stroll Every Half Hour," 2023).

Remember, movement is exercise, even at low intensity. Housework, gardening, walking the dog, dancing in your kitchen, playing with kids, taking the stairs, it all contributes to your fitness and well-being. Everyday activities can burn as many calories as a gym session. Many women become more sedentary during menopause, either because of busy schedules or fatigue from symptoms. But fighting that inertia with frequent movement can make a tremendous difference.

For example, park a bit farther from the store or do gentle stretches while watching TV. Over time, these habits become an effortless part of your life. You'll likely notice you feel less stiff and more energetic on days when you include plenty of natural movement.

Small Ways to Move More Each Day

Think of these as simple "movement snacks" you can weave into daily life. They do not require planning, equipment, or extra time. They are just little choices that keep your body from staying still too long.

Stand and Stretch

If you have been sitting for a while, stand up and take a quick walk around the room or do ten squats. Little by little, you will be teaching your body that it is meant to move.

Take Hourly Breaks

Set a timer to stand up at least once an hour. Do a quick stretch, march in place, or walk to the nearest window and back.

Work Walking into Routines

Pace when you are on a phone call, or take a 5-minute stroll at lunch. Park farther from your destination or take the stairs for an easy cardio boost.

Make Chores Active

Fold laundry standing up, scrub the counters with energy, or carry groceries in smaller loads. These moments add up.

Add Music

Put on your favorite songs while tidying up or play tag with your dog. You will build steps and energy without even noticing.

Everyday movement keeps your body limber and your blood circulating. Especially during menopause, consistency is more important than intensity. Ten 1-minute bursts of movement spread throughout the day can be as beneficial as one continuous 10-minute walk. Give yourself permission to value all of the movement activities you do. It all counts toward a healthier, more energetic you.

Smarter, Not Harder

For many years, "cardio" (aerobic exercise that raises your heart rate) was the go-to for fitness. Then some claimed that women over forty should avoid cardio because it can raise stress hormones. The truth lies in balance. Cardio is not the enemy. In fact, done wisely, it can be a powerful ally for your heart, mood, and metabolism. The key is to approach it in a smart, hormone-informed way.

Let's dispel the myth that "cardio is bad for your hormones." It's an oversimplification. Excessive high-intensity cardio, like intense workouts without enough rest, can spike cortisol (the stress hormone). That isn't helpful, especially if you're already stressed or sleep-deprived. For example, a long, hard run on an empty stomach might leave you exhausted.

However, that doesn't mean all aerobic exercise is off the table. Moderate cardio, especially in short bursts, has many benefits. It improves your insulin sensitivity (helping your body manage blood sugar). It supports your mitochondria, the energy powerhouses in your cells. It boosts your mood with a surge of endorphins. And it can even help you sleep better at night.

What does "smart" midlife cardio look like? It means focusing on moderate-intensity activities that feel good. For example, take a brisk walk in the fresh air, enjoy a casual bike ride, swim laps at a comfortable pace, or do a fun dance fitness video in your living room. You might choose a Sunday morning bike ride with a friend or take two brisk walks during your workdays. Even 5–10 minutes of getting your heart rate up can yield "big gains in metabolic health," according to experts. A short power walk around the block or a quick dance session can lift your mood and get your blood flowing. You might set a goal to jog in place or do jumping jacks in the afternoon when you hit a work slump. These mini sessions can reliably boost your energy and clear your mind.

Listen to your body's cues. Being "cardio smart" also means matching your workouts to the right timing and ensuring proper recovery. If you feel anxious or haven't slept well (common during menopause), a long, intense cardio session might not be what your body needs that day. Shorter intervals can often be better than long workouts, since prolonged exercise can drive cortisol up and potentially hinder your progress. For example, you might do twenty minutes of alternating fast and slow walking, or mix light aerobics with strength moves. This way you get the cardiovascular benefits without overtaxing your system.

Be sure to include recovery. Try to vary your cardio intensity throughout the week. For example, do moderate effort on two or three days, include some higher-intensity bursts on one day, and have a couple of lighter or rest days. This pattern respects the natural energy rhythms of midlife. Also, consider doing cardio after you have eaten (a meal or snack). You'll feel better and avoid spiking stress hormones from exercising on low blood sugar. Stay hydrated and cool down after exercise, especially if you're prone to hot flashes.

When done right, cardio can be a joy. It strengthens your heart and lungs, helps burn calories and manage weight, and is one of the best mood boosters around. During menopause, when the risk of cardiovascular disease goes up, staying aerobically active becomes even more important for protecting your heart. Many women also find that a good sweat is a great stress reliever. Aerobic exercise triggers the release of serotonin and dopamine, brain chemicals that make you feel happier and calmer.

A moderate, enjoyable cardio routine a few times a week, combined with your daily movement snacks and strength training, will round out your fitness in a balanced way. Find something you enjoy, keep it manageable, and remember that consistency matters more than intensity. Your heart, your waistline, and even your hormones will thank you.

Rebuilding Dynamic Movement

Think about hopping over a puddle, dashing across a street, or catching yourself if you trip. These quick, dynamic movements (essentially power and agility) are abilities we often lose as we get older. When we stop jumping, we start to lose the fast-twitch muscle fibers that give us spring and speed. This "jump decline" isn't obvious at first. Then one day you might stumble on an uneven sidewalk and notice your reaction time isn't what it used to be. Or you try to jog across the road and feel oddly uncoordinated.

So why do many women stop doing dynamic, bouncy movements? Some of it is cultural. We get the message that running, jumping, or playful "silly" moves are for the young. We might also fear injuring ourselves, looking foolish, or (very commonly if you have a weak pelvic floor) fear leaking urine when jumping or running. These concerns often lead women to stick to gentler, straight-line motions and avoid impact. But avoiding dynamic movement actually speeds up the decline in our ability to do those movements.

The less you jump, the more your body "forgets" how. Your muscles and connective tissues lose elasticity. The good news is you can safely retrain your body for power, agility, and even a stronger pelvic floor. Start building pelvic floor strength with gentle jumping, Kegel exercises, and yoga poses like Bridge pose or Goddess pose. These exercises train those muscles to handle pressure and can improve urinary incontinence.

Lena, age 47, realized one day that she hadn't run or jumped in years. She was an avid walker but avoided anything high-impact. When her teenage daughter challenged her to a short sprint, Lena hesitated. She felt clumsy and worried she might twist an ankle or embarrass herself. That was a wake-up call. Lena decided to rebuild her agility. She started in her living room with something simple: hopping in place.

Over the next few weeks, she moved up to a beginner rebounding workout on a mini trampoline. It was easier on her joints but still gave her that springy feeling. She also practiced side-to-side steps and quick toe taps during her favorite TV show. A couple of months later, Lena reported that she could sprint to catch the bus without worry. She also felt more confident in her body. "I didn't realize how much I missed moving fast," she says. "It's like I reclaimed a bit of my youth, and my body trusts itself again."

You can start small to rebuild dynamic movement, and gently reawaken those fast-twitch fibers. Here are some ideas to safely get your bounce back:

Begin With Ankle Hops or Rebounding

For ankle hops, stand near a wall or chair for support and do mini vertical jumps, just lift your heels and bounce up an inch or two in place. Or use a mini trampoline (rebounder) if you have one. It's a low-impact way to practice jumping without jarring your joints.

Progress to Slightly Bigger Moves

After you're comfortable with gentle hops, you can retrain your muscles to absorb impact with bigger motions. For example, use an exercise step platform and quickly tap one foot then the other on it (as if running in place). Or step off a low platform and land in a squat.

Move in Different Directions

Don't just move forward—include side-to-side motions to build hip and pelvic stability. Side shuffles, grapevine steps, or Zumba moves are fun dynamic movements that also get your heart rate up.

Play Like a Kid

Games like hopscotch, jump rope, or tag all sneak in dynamic movement that builds fast-twitch muscles.

Adding jumping and quick movements to your workouts pays off in everyday life. Quick, powerful muscle actions can help prevent falls or help you catch yourself if you trip. This is a major factor in staying safe and independent as you age. Studies show that building fast-twitch muscle power is very effective for preventing falls in older adults. Dynamic movement training also has hidden benefits: it challenges your brain and nervous system. Learning a new coordination pattern (like a side shuffle or a ladder drill) is brain training as much as body training. It creates new neural pathways and wakes up your proprioception (your sense of your body's position and movement in space). Many women say that agility training makes them feel sharper and more youthful.

Challenge yourself to reawaken your confidence in quick movements and have fun with it. Add a bit of youthful play to your routine. In the process, you'll make your body more capable and resilient.

Reclaiming Ease and Freedom in Your Body

Many women in menopause experience aching joints and stiffness. This often comes from long hours of sitting, repetitive routines, and hormonal shifts that affect tissues. The good news is you can greatly improve your mobility with simple practices that use your body's full range of motion. Mobility is not just about touching your toes (that's flexibility). Mobility means being able to use that flexibility in real life, like squatting down, twisting to reach something in the backseat of the car, or getting up off the floor without using your hands. Mobility is as much about strength and coordination as it is about flexibility.

Why does mobility tend to decrease in menopause? One reason is the drop in estrogen. Estrogen helps keep joints and connective tissue supple. When estrogen declines, there is less joint lubrication, and tendons and ligaments lose collagen (so they feel tighter). Muscle recovery also slows down. On top of that, if you're more sedentary because of work or fatigue, your fascia (connective tissue) can develop adhesions. You also lose the variety of movement that keeps you limber.

Joint pain and stiffness are very common in perimenopause. Up to 50% of women report these symptoms in the hips, spine, neck, and shoulders (Shapcott, 2024). There is a paradox: when you feel stiff, the last thing you want to do is move, yet movement is exactly what will help you feel better. As physical therapist Kristen Gasnick explains, movement lubricates your joints by circulating synovial fluid (the nourishing fluid in your joint capsules). Every time you gently stretch, rotate, or bend, you flush out old fluid and bring in fresh nutrients to your cartilage.

Mobility exercises also strengthen the muscles around your joints, easing the load on them and providing stability. Over time, this can delay or reduce arthritis symptoms. Beyond the physical benefits, mobility exercises can also reset your nervous system.

Slow, gentle movements combined with deep breathing (like in yoga) trigger a relaxation response. This reduces anxiety and improves mood. As your body starts to loosen up, you stand taller, feel more youthful, and breathe more easily.

Joint-Friendly Strength

Joint pain can make the very thought of exercise daunting. When your knees, hips, or back hurt, resting on the couch feels more appealing than a workout. Many women in midlife avoid movement for fear of worsening the pain. The paradox is that the right kind of movement can actually relieve joint pain. In fact, research shows that moving more is one of the best ways to ease achy joints. Regular, gentle exercise helps reduce pain and stiffness. It might be the last thing you feel like doing when you're achy. But even a little movement sends blood flow to your joints, lubricates them, and releases the endorphins that act like natural painkillers.

Midlife isn't a decline. It's an upgrade if you train for it. Building muscle can stabilize and safeguard your joints. When your muscles and tendons are strong, they absorb more of the strain so your joints don't have to. Resistance or weight training is especially helpful. Strength training not only rebuilds muscle (since muscle loss accelerates in menopause) but it also improves bone density and joint stability. Over time, this can mean fewer injuries and a lot less pain. Women who include strength training in their routine often report reduced arthritis symptoms and better mobility. Studies even suggest a long-term benefit. Older adults who did regular strength training had significantly lower rates of knee osteoarthritis and pain compared to those who never lifted weights (Ho et al., 2023). And it's never too late to start. Even people who begin strength exercises after age fifty see protective benefits similar to those who started exercising earlier.

High-impact workouts or intense routines aren't necessary (and can be counterproductive if they flare up your pain). Instead, opt for low-impact, gentle movement that gets you moving without pounding your joints. Yoga or Tai Chi are great options: they focus on flexibility, balance, and muscle engagement with minimal joint strain. The important thing is consistency, not intensity. Aiming for even 10–15 minutes of movement daily will start to build your strength and reduce stiffness. As your comfort improves, you can gradually step it up. Maybe you start with a short neighborhood walk. Over time, you might find you can go further or add in light weight training or a dance class. Each session helps lubricate your joints and maintain your range of motion.

Exercise not only eases joint pain by keeping the joints supple, it also helps control weight (extra pounds put more pressure on joints) and releases stress. Many women discover that as they build muscle, their posture and balance improve. This reduces joint strain and the risk of falls. It's a positive feedback loop: move a little, feel a little better, which lets you move a little more. Over a few months, these small steps can lead to major improvements in strength and confidence.

So how can you improve mobility? A few gentle movement practices are especially well-suited for midlife women:

Pilates

Pilates is a form of exercise focused on core strength, controlled movements, and alignment. It strengthens the spine, hips, and core without high impact. Pilates can improve your posture and muscle balance, which in turn corrects faulty movement patterns that lead to chronic strain (especially in the knees, hips, and lower back). It's also excellent for strengthening the abdominal and pelvic floor muscles.

Wall Pilates

Wall Pilates involves Pilates-inspired exercises you perform while standing or lying with your feet or hands pressing against a wall. It's great for beginners or people with vertigo or joint issues. For example, you might do a wall squat or a leg lift with your back flat against the wall. The wall helps ensure you're using the right form and provides support. It's low-impact and accessible, yet it still builds strength in your entire body (especially the glutes, legs, and core, which are crucial for stability).

Yoga

Yoga has been shown to improve balance and flexibility. Some studies also found it can reduce menopause symptoms like sleep disturbances and mood swings. Certain styles, like yin yoga, focus on slow movements and holding poses to release deep tension. Other styles, like hatha or vinyasa, build heat and flexibility through more movement. Even a simple practice with a few key stretches (like cat-cow spinal stretches, a couple of downward dogs, and some hip openers) can serve as a "nervous system reset," unclenching tight muscles and lowering stress hormones. One of yoga's hidden gifts is that it teaches you to breathe through discomfort and practice mind-body awareness.

Stretching

Regular gentle stretching combats stiffness and helps you unwind in a calm way. For example, you might slowly roll your neck and shoulders, do some gentle torso twists, stretch out your calves and hamstrings, touch your toes and stretch your back, practice some hip openers, and then do wrist and ankle circles.

Each of these practices can be adapted for anybody. When done regularly, they work wonders to improve your mobility, posture, and energy.

Finally, let's talk about the emotional side of mobility. When your body moves freely, it directly impacts your mood. We often hold stress and emotions as tension in our bodies and releasing that tension through movement can be very healing. Mobility work teaches patience and self-compassion, because when you learn to breathe through a stretch, you build trust in your body. Many women say they feel calmer, more grounded, and more optimistic after a gentle mobility session. Stretching can lower cortisol and increase relaxation responses.

How to Start Gentle, Doable Habits

Starting a mobility practice might feel daunting if you're very stiff or out of practice, but it's easy to begin with a few gentle habits:

3-minute Evening Stretch Flow

End each day with a bedtime routine to release tension. For example, slowly tilt your head side to side and do some shoulder rolls. Clasp your hands behind your back for a chest-opening stretch. Gently bend forward and place your hands on your shins to stretch your hamstrings. You can finish with a pigeon pose or a gentle spinal twist. These simple stretches help reset your nervous system, and send a signal to your body that it's time to relax.

Wall Pilates Once or Twice A Week

Practice a short wall Pilates session focused on core strength and balance. Try wall push-ups, wall-assisted leg lifts, or a wall sit to wake up your deep core muscles. Over time, this will improve your posture and stability.

Morning Cat-Cow

Start your day with a few gentle cat-cow stretches on the floor (to mobilize your spine and hips). Then add a downward dog pose to stretch your calves, hamstrings, and back.

By integrating these small habits, you'll gradually build a sustainable mobility routine. Remember, the goal is to feel good in your body. Be gentle and consistent and listen to your body's cues. On days when you're achy, do extra light stretching. On days when you feel great, enjoy a more active yoga flow or a longer Pilates session.

As you embrace daily movement, smart cardio, dynamic exercise, and mobility work, you are creating a movement-rich lifestyle that will carry you through menopause and beyond. It's about honoring your body with regular, joyful motion. One day it might be a power walk, another day it might be fifteen minutes of Pilates, or dancing in your kitchen and then stretching before bed. It all counts, and it all helps you reconnect with a sense of vitality. The more you move, the more you'll trust your body,and the more you trust your body, the more you'll want to move it.

it might be a ten-minute power walk, another day 15 minutes of Pilates, another day dancing in your kitchen and stretching before bed. It all counts, and it all helps reconnect you with a sense of vitality. The more you move, the more you'll trust your body; the more you trust your body, the more you'll want to move it.

Movement Stacks for Daily Life

Making movement a sustainable habit is easiest when you embed it into what you already do. Instead of viewing exercise as all-or-nothing, think of it as something you layer into your day in small doses.

A movement stack means pairing a small physical action—a brief exercise or stretch—with an existing daily habit. This idea builds on the behavioral science concept of habit stacking. Habit stacking involves linking a new behavior to an established routine so you are more likely to stick with it.

For example, if you always brew coffee in the morning, you could attach a one-minute stretch routine to that habit. By pairing movement with something you are already doing, you reduce friction and build consistency. Your current habits act like anchors. By attaching an exercise to them, you create a reliable cue that makes the new habit automatic.

Everyday Examples

Movement stacks are small, deliberate pairings of activity with something you already do. They create consistency because the cue is built into your routine.

- **Desk Reset**: After sending an email, do a few shoulder rolls or wall angels to ease stiffness.

- **Between Tasks**: Between meetings, try ten squats or a short walk around the building to re-energize.

- **Evening Wind-Down**: Pair your bedtime routine with a gentle spinal twist or a forward fold to signal rest.

- **Short Bursts**: Take a 10-minute brisk walk (or two 5-minute walks), then follow with gentle stretches.

- **Mini Circuit**: Do a 10-minute bodyweight circuit such as squats, modified push-ups, lunges, and a plank.

- **Cardio Boost**: Try five minutes of jumping jacks or stair climbing, then five minutes of fast walking.

- **Go Longer When You Can**: Include bigger activities when possible, such as a weekend hike, bike ride, or nature walk.

Stack your movement sessions throughout the week like building blocks. Swap activities or adjust as needed to fit your schedule. Aim for some movement on most days.

As the CDC's physical activity guidelines say, "Some physical activity is better than none. Adults who sit less and do any amount of moderate-intensity activity gain some health benefits." In short: do what you can, whenever you can. It is always better than an all-or-nothing approach.

Tips for Staying Consistent

Building a lasting habit of movement is all about consistency and positive reinforcement. Here are a few simple strategies to help you stay on track:

- **Track Your Streaks**. Use a calendar, journal, or habit-tracking app to mark each day you did some movement. Seeing a streak of active days can be motivating!

- **Celebrate Small Wins**. Give yourself credit for every action, no matter how small. Did you take a 10-minute walk every day this week? High five! Treat yourself to something enjoyable and healthy for positive reinforcement.

- **Pair Movement With Rewards**. Make your movement time enjoyable by pairing it with something you love. For example, only listen to your favorite podcast when you're out walking, so you'll look forward to your walks.

- **Have a Fallback Plan**. Prepare an ultra-simple, bare-minimum plan for busy days. For instance, if all else fails, do ten crunches before the end of the day. Even if everything else goes off track, that one little action means you're still in the game.

Finally, be kind to yourself: some days you'll do more, other days less. What matters is that you keep showing up. When you stack healthy habits onto your daily routine, you create a sustainable rhythm of activity. Over time, you'll likely find you have more energy, better mood, and a growing confidence in your body.

Do This Today

Sometimes the hardest part is just getting started, especially when it comes to getting your body in motion. You might need to overcome inertia. If you've been inactive, your body tends to stay inactive. Remember Newton's first law of motion: an object at rest stays at rest unless acted upon by an outside force. So be that force: get your body moving, today, right now. Go!

Reflection

How can you help yourself stay consistent with the changes you want to integrate into your daily routine?

Chapter 6
Burnout and Restoration

———

"Burnout happens not from doing too much but from doing too much of what drains you."

Dr. Saundra Dalton Smith, *Sacred Rest*

———

You wake up drenched in sweat and exhausted again. By midday, the slump hits, the brain fog, the urge to nap. Midlife hormonal shifts, especially during perimenopause and menopause, can throw your internal thermostat and energy systems off balance. The result? Hot flashes, night sweats, flushed skin, mood swings, and energy crashes that leave you feeling burned out.

When your physical energy fluctuates dramatically, your mental energy suffers too. If you're feeling depleted, you're not alone. Many women share this experience. The good news is that a few simple, science-backed tactics can help smooth out these ups and downs and restore a steadier sense of energy.

"Menopause hit me like a freight train," Amanda recalls. "Hot flashes, joint pain, sleep disruption, and zero energy. I used to walk 10,000 steps a day. I was barely hitting 1,000. I felt like I was disappearing inside my own body." Doctors told her everything looked fine, and her lab results were normal. But she knew something was off. She felt exhausted, disconnected, and desperate for change.

Hot Flashes and Night Sweats

Hot flashes happen when shifting estrogen levels make your body's thermostat, the hypothalamus, more sensitive. Even a small change in temperature can be misread as overheating, which triggers your body's cooling response: a sudden, intense wave of heat. Research by Thurston (2013) shows that as estrogen fluctuates, the hypothalamus becomes more reactive, leading to these sudden surges.

Hot flashes can strike anytime—at your desk, during exercise, or in the middle of the night when you most need rest.

Dehydration from all that sweating and the drastic energy swings can add to low stamina and brain fog. In other words, all these symptoms can create a vicious cycle that drains your energy. Often, it means you are hormonally overheated, under-rested, and overextended. But routines that include rest, recovery, and proactive moderation can make a difference.

Hot flashes and night sweats aren't just due to hormones; they also involve your sympathetic nervous system (the fight-or-flight system). When the hypothalamus thinks you're too warm, the sympathetic system kicks in. It causes blood vessels to dilate, increasing blood flow to the skin's surface. That leads to the hot, flushed feeling of a hot flash. This response can also activate your sweat glands, which is why a hot flash is often followed by sweating (especially at night). Your body is trying to cool down quickly, which results in those night sweats.

Several lifestyle and environmental factors can make hot flashes and night sweats more intense. Research suggests that alcohol and caffeine can increase the frequency of hot flashes, because they raise heart rate and dilate blood vessels (mimicking your body's hot flash reaction) (Kandiah, 2010). Stress can also raise cortisol, which disrupts hormonal balance. A 2016 study in *Menopause* found that women under high stress had more frequent hot flashes than those with lower stress. In short, stress hormones can make hot flashes feel more intense.

Your body's organs have circadian rhythms, natural biological clocks influenced by light and dark, movement, nutrition, stress, and hormone levels (like estrogen and progesterone). A hormonal imbalance can make it harder for your body to regulate temperature during sleep, leading to night sweats. Night sweats often disrupt sleep, and that links to another hormone issue. As estrogen levels drop, your production of melatonin (the hormone that regulates sleep-wake cycles) also drops. Less melatonin can disrupt your sleep patterns, making it harder to fall or stay asleep. A study by Carpenter et al. (2018) found that women with sleep disturbances also had a higher incidence of hot flashes and night sweats.

These overlapping symptoms can really exhaust you. The good news is that finding relief can help on multiple levels. Try to identify any specific triggers, like stress or heat. Also, avoiding smoking, alcohol, caffeine, and spicy food can be a good start.

Hot flashes and night sweats often come in cycles. In perimenopause, you might first see an increase in hot flashes that eventually peak and then decline as your body adjusts. Research by Freeman (2015) found that hot flashes can last anywhere from a few months to several years, depending on your unique hormonal changes and lifestyle. Some women have occasional flashes, while others face persistent episodes. This variability highlights the complexity of menopause and how individual the experience can be.

Cooling Techniques

Temperature regulation during sleep is crucial for hormonal balance and energy restoration.
Dr. Sara Gottfried, The Hormone Cure

To help your body stay cool at night, lower the thermostat and use breathable cotton or bamboo sheets. You might also try a fan, a cooling pillow, or cooling pajamas made from natural fibers like bamboo, hemp, or eucalyptus. Stay hydrated during the day to help regulate your body temperature. Consider adding electrolytes like magnesium and potassium to your water. Drink iced herbal teas (such as peppermint or sage) and avoid caffeine and alcohol.

Cooling Breath Exercise: The yoga breathing practice, Sitali Pranayama, has been shown to reduce body temperature and stress levels (Sengupta, 2012). To practice Sitali Pranayama, roll your tongue (or purse your lips if you can't roll your tongue) and inhale slowly as if sipping air through a straw. Then exhale through your nose. Repeat this for two or three minutes.

Fatigue

*When energy flags, you don't need more hustle
you need more oxygen, light, and calm.*
Dr. Aviva Romm, Hormone Intelligence

As estrogen and progesterone fall, cortisol can rise, leading to "wired at night, tired in the morning" cycles (Prior, 2010). Meanwhile, your mitochondria (the energy producers in cells) become less efficient with age and hormonal shifts. That means cellular functions like tissue repair and energy regulation slow down. The result is less energy production, even if you're eating and sleeping well. Many women find themselves stuck in a cycle of fatigue that goes beyond normal sleep issues. It's easy to blame hot flashes and night sweats for your exhaustion. But in truth, your hormones play a major role in how tired you feel throughout the day.

When estrogen dips, it can lower your serotonin levels (serotonin is your brain's "feel-good" neurotransmitter). Low serotonin means lower energy, mood swings, and sometimes feelings of sadness or depression. All of that adds to your fatigue. Then there's progesterone, the hormone that calms your mind and helps you sleep. When progesterone levels drop (as they do during menopause), it becomes much harder to wind down at night. You might find yourself tossing and turning instead of getting restful sleep. If your body feels more "on edge," it's a sign that it's missing this hormonal balance.

Thyroid health is another factor in your energy levels. The thyroid regulates metabolism, so if it's out of sync you may feel sluggish or struggle with daily tasks. Some women, especially during menopause, experience mild thyroid issues that add to fatigue. If your fatigue is persistent and doesn't improve with lifestyle changes, talk to your healthcare provider. Sometimes addressing thyroid imbalances or other health issues can make a big difference.

During menopause, you're likely dealing with the extra stress of balancing daily responsibilities with physical and emotional changes. High stress can push cortisol into overdrive, making you feel agitated and exhausted at the same time. When cortisol is out of balance, it disrupts your natural energy cycle. You might feel wiped out in the morning but then wired late at night. It's a vicious cycle that leaves you drained, no matter how many hours you spend in bed. A few practical habits can help break this cycle. Focus on restoring your natural circadian rhythm, reducing stress, practicing good sleep hygiene, and nourishing your body. Together, these steps can help bring a sense of balance back to your daily life.

Amy found herself struggling to keep up with her daily routine. She would wake at 3 a.m. with her mind racing, and by afternoon she would crash with fatigue. She started using mindful breathing techniques to reduce stress. She switched to an anti-inflammatory diet and focused on eating plenty of nutrient-dense whole foods. She also added probiotics and GABA and L-theanine supplements to help with sleep and anxiety. Over time, Amy felt more balanced and resilient. Her sleep quality improved at night, and her energy leveled out during the day.

Break the Cycle of Fatigue

Here are a few steps to start balancing your hormones and address factors that contribute to fatigue:

Sunlight First Thing. When you absorb morning light, it helps reset your circadian rhythm, lower melatonin, and jump-start energy and focus.

Manage Stress. Find ways to lower your stress and regulate your cortisol levels. This can include regular mindfulness practices, journaling, or spending time in nature.

Practice Good Sleep Hygiene. Stick to a consistent sleep schedule, create a restorative wind-down routine, make your bedroom a sleep sanctuary (dark, cool, quiet), and avoid eating or drinking alcohol late in the evening.

Nourish Your Body. Drink plenty of water and eat balanced meals with fresh fruit, vegetables, lean protein, and whole grains to stabilize blood sugar and fuel your body.

Exercise Regularly. Physical activity, particularly light to moderate exercise, can boost energy levels and regulate hormone production. Try a brisk walk in the morning or a yoga session before bed to help improve sleep quality and energy.

By taking this holistic approach and addressing the roots of your fatigue, you can reclaim your energy. Focus on real food, hydration, mindfulness, movement, and joyful habits to protect your mood.

Rethink What Renews You

A good day starts with a calm night and a calm night begins with small choices.
Arianna Huffington, *The Sleep Revolution*

Pay attention to habits that might be draining your energy and try to replace them with healthier ones. For example, having alcohol in the evening might seem relaxing, but it disrupts sleep stages and can worsen hot flashes (Freeman et al., 2015). In the past you might have had wine at night with no issues, but now it could be affecting you. You might notice you wake up in the middle of the night feeling dehydrated, or that alcohol is affecting your mood and digestion.

High-carb foods can cause a rapid blood sugar spike followed by a crash, leading to irritability and exhaustion. Very intense cardio routines can also push your cortisol levels up. In menopause, less can be more. Try adjusting your daily routine with a bit more moderation in areas where you might be pushing your body too hard.

10-Minute Routines

Here are some sample 10-minute routines for different times of day:

Morning (Hydration, movement, and light to regulate your biological clock)

- Wake up and drink water.
- Step outside for natural sunlight (even on cloudy days).
- Move your body (take a brisk walk, do some stretching, or lift weights).
- Eat a protein-rich breakfast (like eggs, yogurt, or a smoothie).

Afternoon (When you feel an afternoon crash, tend to your physical needs)

- Drink a tall glass of water with a pinch of sea salt and a squeeze of lemon.
- Take a walk outside in the sunlight.
- Add protein to your next snack.

Bedtime (Hydration, relaxation, and mindful light reduction to soothe body and mind)

- Dim the lights, have a glass of water or a cup of herbal tea, and take a magnesium supplement about an hour before bed.
- Try a little cold therapy: place an ice pack on the side of your neck (below your ears) to stimulate the vagus nerve.
- Do something restorative like gentle yoga or write in your journal before bed.

Charlotte, a high school counselor and mother of two teenagers, started waking up at 3 a.m. drenched in sweat, heart pounding, mind racing. Her energy would tank by 2 p.m. each day. She'd grab a muffin and coffee hoping for a boost but would just crash harder by dinner.

"I felt like I was melting down... literally and emotionally," she says. "Even the smallest things started overwhelming me." On a friend's suggestion, Charlotte tried two small changes: she sipped an electrolyte drink first thing in the morning, and she set a timer for a 10-minute walk right after lunch. She also switched to cooling sheets and kept a spray bottle in the fridge, misting her neck and chest before bed. It became a simple, soothing ritual.

At first, it didn't feel like much, the walk was short and the heat still came in waves. But she noticed something started to change. "By the end of that first week, I realized I wasn't dreading the nights so much," Charlotte says. "The sweats still came, but I was sleeping deeper. My mind wasn't foggy. I had more room inside myself. More calm."

Do This Today

Take ten minutes to do something relaxing. You might:

- Touch your toes and stretch your spine.
- Drink a glass of lemon water.
- Eat some fresh fruit.
- Walk barefoot outside and soak up natural light.
- Try cold therapy by placing an ice pack on your neck to stimulate the vagus nerve and reduce hot flashes.

Reflection

Think about what brings you a sense of peace. Is it spending a few minutes tending to your garden, reading for pleasure, or singing? How might you find a small pocket of time to do it more often?

Chapter 7
Intimacy and Pleasure

———

"Menopause has always been painted as the end of your sexual era... but in reality, it can be a profoundly liberating period of sexual self-determination."

Leslie Morgan

———

If you've noticed sex feels different lately, this is a common experience. Many women in midlife find that intimacy shifts during menopause, sometimes in challenging ways, such as vaginal dryness or an unpredictable libido, and this can spark worries about the future of their sex lives (Sarmento et al., 2021). Culturally, we've been fed the myth that menopause is the death of desire, but your sexuality doesn't end with menopause. In fact, for many women, this life stage becomes a time to redefine pleasure on their own terms.

Your sexuality doesn't end with menopause.

Yes, your body is changing. But with a little knowledge, practical tools, and self-compassion, you can continue to have a satisfying, meaningful intimate life. We'll speak candidly about the physical changes that can affect sex, the emotional and relationship dimensions of midlife intimacy, and the many ways you can nurture comfort and connection in the bedroom and beyond. Consider this a reassuring guide to embracing your sexual well-being during menopause, and a reminder that you deserve pleasure and closeness just as much as ever.

The Physical Changes That Affect Intimacy

One of the most common midlife complaints is vaginal dryness. As estrogen levels fall during menopause, the tissues of the vagina thin out and produce far less natural moisture. The vaginal walls become less elastic and more delicate. You might find that sex which used to be pleasurable now feels irritating or even painful because of this dryness and fragility. About three out of four postmenopausal women experience symptoms of vaginal dryness or atrophy (Sarmento et al., 2021). The technical term for these changes is genitourinary syndrome of menopause (GSM). GSM can include dryness, increased urinary urgency, and more frequent UTIs. However, the hallmark symptom most women notice is the lack of lubrication that leads to discomfort or painful intercourse.

These changes happen because estrogen was the hormone that kept your vaginal lining thick and well lubricated. Without enough estrogen, the tissue gets thinner, and the vagina can actually become shorter and narrower. Less estrogen also means less blood flow to the genitals, which can affect how easily you become aroused. The clitoris, another estrogen-sensitive organ, may get less blood flow and stimulation, which can make it a bit less sensitive than before. In practical terms, you might find it takes longer to get turned on. You may need more direct stimulation to reach orgasm, or your orgasms might feel different (perhaps milder, or they take more time and effort). All of this is a normal result of the hormonal shifts happening in your body.

Another physical factor is libido fluctuation. It's common for women to report that their desire for sex diminishes or becomes erratic in midlife. About 40–50% of women going through menopause experience a noticeable drop in sex drive (Scavello et al., 2019). Some days you might feel zero interest, while other times intimacy still sounds appealing. Hormones play a role here: declining estrogen (and the small amount of testosterone women produce) can subtly dial down your "drive."

Intimacy is yours to define.

It's worth noting that not every woman has less desire at this stage. Some women actually feel freer and more sexual than ever once they're past the worry of pregnancy and feel less inhibited by others' opinions. Some feel sexier when they take time to redefine their style and find clothes that make them feel body-positive and confident. There's a wide range of "normal" in midlife libido. The key is understanding the changes your body is going through. That way, you can address any problems (like dryness, pain, low energy, or lack of confidence) that might be dampening your desire.

The Emotional and Relational Dimensions

Menopause often coincides with many life changes that can affect intimacy. You might be juggling kids, caring for aging parents, or facing changes in your career. You might be dating again after a divorce, or in a long-term marriage that's adapting to empty-nest life. All these changes can influence your sexual rhythm.

Stress, whether from workload, caregiving, or relationship issues, can really dampen libido. As relationship expert Esther Perel writes in *Mating in Captivity*, "It's hard to experience desire when you're weighed down by concern."

On an emotional level, many women struggle with body image and self-esteem in midlife. As estrogen declines, it's common to gain weight or notice your body's shape changing (often in unwelcome ways). If you feel self-conscious, you might avoid sexual situations because you worry about how you look to your partner. Plus, mood shifts are common in perimenopause, increased irritability, anxiety, or bouts of depression aren't unusual. It's hard to feel in the mood for love if you're feeling blue or on edge. And if you're taking an antidepressant for your mood, those medications can sometimes lower libido as a side effect.

Relationships evolve at midlife too. If you have a partner, they may be going through their own health or hormonal changes (for example, a male partner might have erectile difficulties or lower testosterone). This can create a mismatch in arousal or ability that requires patience and understanding on both sides. Long-term couples might also fall into routines that feel stale, or there may be unspoken resentments that dampen the spark.

Emotional intimacy is just as important as physical connection.

On the other hand, some couples find a new emotional closeness as they age, especially once the kids are grown and they have more time for each other again. Emotional intimacy, feeling heard, loved, and connected, is deeply linked to sexual intimacy. In fact, studies show that feeling emotionally supported by your partner is a key predictor of sexual satisfaction in midlife. If you feel disconnected or unseen outside the bedroom, you'll often have less interest in intimacy inside the bedroom. That's why open communication is so crucial during this life phase.

Arousal and Pleasure

Let's talk more about hormones and sexual response, because it can be hard to tell what's physical versus emotional. As mentioned earlier, falling estrogen levels directly affect your genital tissues. Less estrogen means less blood flow to the vagina and clitoris. This can mean you need more time and stimulation to become aroused. For example, maybe you used to get naturally lubricated after just a few passionate kisses. Now your body might respond more slowly, lubrication might only happen after extended foreplay, or you may need to use a lubricant.

Orgasms can change too. Some women say their orgasms aren't as intense or are harder to reach after menopause. Lower estrogen and testosterone can be partly responsible, since hormone receptors in the brain and nerves influence orgasmic response. If vaginal tissues are drier or thinner, the sensations during intercourse might be weaker than before. Orgasms can also trigger hot flashes, which can be distracting during intimacy. However, it's absolutely possible to continue having orgasms (even multiple ones) in midlife. In fact, some women have the most intense orgasms of their lives once they learn what pleases them. Physically, an orgasm is a reflex of the pelvic floor muscles contracting rhythmically. Healthy pelvic muscles and good blood flow are key to strong orgasms. So while hormones set the stage, other factors like muscle tone, circulation, and technique are just as important.

You may also notice that sexual desire shows up differently now than it did when you were younger. Many women in midlife shift from what's called spontaneous desire (feeling turned on out of the blue or from a fantasy) to more of a responsive desire model. Responsive desire means you might only feel "in the mood" after sexual activity has started. For example, you might rarely actively crave sex on your own. But if your partner initiates cuddling or you start fooling around, you realize you do feel desire once things get going. You haven't "lost" your libido, it's just operating more subtly now.

Knowing this can actually be liberating. You might choose to initiate intimacy or agree to sexual play before you feel a strong desire, trusting that your body will catch up once arousal begins. As sex educator Emily Nagoski explains, we need to let go of the myth of the sexual "spark," the idea that desire must strike like lightning for sex to be worthwhile. In midlife, desire often needs to be cultivated, like gently coaxing a flame, and that's okay! It might mean scheduling intimate time or creating more deliberate romantic scenarios to set the mood. It can also help to educate yourself about sex through books, guides, or podcasts. There is a lot more open conversation about sexual pleasure and intimacy these days, which can help you discover new kinds of enjoyment and new ways to connect with yourself and your partner. This is where communication and experimentation become really important.

Tools and Treatments for Comfort and Pleasure

There are many tools and treatments to help with the physical challenges of midlife sex. You don't have to "just live with" painful dryness or a dwindling libido. A combination of modern medicine and some old-fashioned creativity can make a world of difference. Let's start with the basics.

Vaginal Moisturizers and Lubricants

These over-the-counter helpers are often the first line of defense against dryness. A little extra moisture can restore a lot of enjoyment. Lubricants and moisturizers are related, but slightly different. A vaginal moisturizer is used more like a routine treatment, you apply it every few days (even when you're not having sex) to hydrate the vaginal tissues and improve overall moisture. Many women find that using a moisturizer regularly (some contain hyaluronic acid or other soothing ingredients) helps their vagina feel more comfortable day to day. A lubricant is a product you apply right before or during sex to reduce friction and increase comfort. There are plenty of options: water-based lubes are very popular and safe with condoms, and silicone-based lubes last longer. There are even oil-based lubes (like coconut or olive oil). Note: If you use latex condoms, avoid oil-based lubes because they can degrade latex. In menopause, lubricant is your friend.

Local Vaginal Estrogen Therapy

One of the most effective remedies for vaginal dryness and atrophy is to put a little estrogen directly where it's needed, in the vagina. Low-dose vaginal estrogen comes as creams, tablets, or a small ring. It can "rescue" thinning vaginal tissue by rebuilding it to a healthier, more supple state. Because the dose is low and applied locally, very little estrogen enters your bloodstream (it mainly stays in the vaginal walls). This means even women who cannot take systemic hormone therapy for medical reasons (for example, some breast cancer survivors) may be cleared by their doctors to use vaginal estrogen safely. After a few weeks of treatment, women often notice that they produce more natural lubrication again, sex stops hurting, and even issues like urinary urgency or recurrent UTIs improve (a healthier vaginal lining helps support the whole urinary tract). If you've been suffering from dryness and over-the-counter lubes aren't enough, talk to your healthcare provider about vaginal estrogen to restore the vaginal environment.

Other Medical Therapies

If vaginal dryness is causing significant discomfort, there are other medical therapies that can help rebuild your comfort. Besides estrogen, there are a couple of newer prescription options. One is **DHEA** (dehydroepiandrosterone), a hormone precursor used as a nightly vaginal suppository. Your body converts DHEA into small amounts of estrogen and androgen locally. This has been shown to ease painful sex and improve vaginal tissue health as well. Another option is an oral medication called **ospemifene** (brand name Osphena). It isn't an estrogen but acts like one in the vaginal tissue to combat thinning and pain. These treatments are usually for women who either can't use estrogen or prefer a pill approach. There is also a non-surgical laser treatment that can help restore vaginal tissues and reduce chronic UTIs and painful intercourse.

Testosterone Therapy

For women who experience a big drop in sexual desire and find it distressing, there are medical options. Some doctors prescribe a low dose of testosterone (usually off-label, since there's no female-specific product in many places). Research shows it can improve sexual desire in postmenopausal women.

The truth is, desire is complex. If vaginal discomfort has been treated and you still feel no libido (and you're unhappy about it), it's worth talking to a provider. But often, improving other factors, like physical comfort, emotional intimacy, and stress levels, will naturally rekindle desire.

Your pelvic floor, the "hammock" of muscles inside your pelvis that supports your bladder, uterus and bowels, can also change. These muscles contract during orgasm and help with vaginal tone and sensation. Menopause and aging can weaken your pelvic floor muscles (just as muscle mass decreases elsewhere), especially if you've had children or pelvic surgery. A weak pelvic floor can lead to less intense orgasms or even incontinence during sex (like a bit of urine leakage at orgasm or penetration). On the other hand, an overly tight pelvic floor (often from holding tension or past pain) can cause painful sex.

Pelvic floor exercises, also known as Kegel exercises (where you squeeze and release those internal muscles), can make a big difference. Strengthening these muscles increases blood flow to the vagina and clitoris, which naturally enhances arousal and lubrication. It can also lead to stronger orgasms (think of it like toning your "orgasm muscle"). If you have pain from tight muscles, a pelvic floor therapist can teach you relaxation techniques or recommend dilators, gentle devices to retrain the vaginal muscles to relax and stretch without pain. Even simple daily Kegels or pelvic-focused yoga moves can help you feel more "in touch" with that area of your body, which can lead to better sexual sensation.

Don't underestimate the impact of general health habits on your sex life. Moving your body, for example, can move your libido. Regular exercise has been shown to boost mood and energy, improve body confidence, and even enhance arousal by improving circulation. Even if you feel tired, getting your blood pumping with a brisk walk, a dance session, or some strength training can spark a positive chain reaction. You'll feel more vibrant and connected to your body, your stress levels drop, and your brain gets a dose of endorphins, all of which set the stage for interest in intimacy. Good sleep also plays an essential role. When you're well-rested, your libido has a much better chance to flourish. Menopause can wreak havoc on sleep (thanks to night sweats and insomnia), so addressing those symptoms (as we discussed in the Better Sleep chapter) can indirectly help your sex life.

Eating a balanced diet and staying hydrated support overall vaginal health too. For instance, some evidence suggests omega-3 fats and vitamin E lead to healthier tissues. And of course, drinking enough water helps all your mucous membranes. Staying hydrated can help with vaginal dryness, and avoiding caffeine and alcohol can also help (since they're diuretics that dry you out). Probiotics, through foods or supplements, can support a healthy balance in your gut and vaginal microbiome, reduce inflammation, and maintain a healthy pH. This can also help ease vaginal dryness.

Lastly, consider stress management as a libido booster. Chronic stress floods your body with cortisol, a libido killer that can also worsen vaginal dryness and fatigue. By nurturing your overall wellness, you create conditions for your sexual self to thrive. Remember, sexuality is mind and body. A healthy heart, mind, and body set the foundation for a healthy sex life.

The Power of Open Conversation

Now that we've covered physical solutions, let's talk about the most important tool of all: communication, both with your partner (if you have one) and with yourself. It's often said that the brain is the biggest sex organ and part of that comes from how we mentally connect (or don't connect) with ourselves and with our partners. Talking openly about what you're experiencing can prevent misunderstandings and deepen your bond. Learning more about yourself and your relationship can help you feel more embodied and connected.

Many of us grew up in a culture where talking about sex felt awkward or taboo. So if it's hard for you to bring up these topics, you're not alone. But midlife can be the perfect time to break that pattern. Start by choosing a good moment. Pick a relaxed time outside the bedroom, when neither of you is rushed or distracted. Frame it as a team effort: it's something to navigate together. If you feel nervous, it's okay to admit that.

Be direct and specific about what's happening with your body and emotions. For example, if vaginal dryness is causing pain, explain that lower estrogen has made things drier and that it hurts without plenty of lubrication. This lets your partner know that you do want to be intimate, but you need to solve the discomfort. Many partners, especially men, may not understand what menopause symptoms feel like. They might misinterpret your wince of pain as lack of interest or think you're pulling away, when in reality you're dealing with physical pain or self-consciousness. By cluing your partner in, you remove the guesswork. Often, a partner's biggest fear is that you're no longer attracted to them. So imagine their relief when they learn it's a solvable issue, like dryness or needing more foreplay.

It's also important to share the emotional changes you're feeling. Let your partner know it's not that they're undesirable, it's that your body and mind are going through a lot. Invite them to share their feelings too. Maybe your partner has fears or confusion they haven't expressed. Creating a safe space for both of you to talk can bring you closer. Women who feel emotionally supported by their partners tend to have better sexual experiences. Even just talking about it can start to relieve anxiety on both sides.

Keep in mind that one conversation won't magically fix everything. Try to check in every so often. Normalize the idea that it's okay to talk about sex regularly, to take the pressure off any single talk. Think of it as a collaborative project where both of you have a say in the pleasure you're creating.

Self-Exploration and Redefining Intimacy

For many women, self-exploration (masturbation) becomes a key part of midlife sexual health. If you've never masturbated much or felt shy about it, consider that now might be the perfect time to start. Masturbation increases blood flow to the genital tissues, which helps keep your vagina more elastic and responsive. Menopause experts often say "use it or lose it," meaning that regular sexual activity, even solo, helps maintain vaginal tone and lubrication.

Exploring yourself can teach you which touches or techniques arouse you. You can then communicate this to your partner. If you don't have a partner right now, it's still important to be honest with yourself about your needs. This is a good time to explore what makes you feel good and become more familiar with the nuances of your changing body and what brings you pleasure. As you learn how your body responds to different fantasies, types of pressure, strokes, stimulation, positions, or even toys, you gain a lot of insight into what pleases you and the kinds of orgasms you can have. This deep personal knowledge means that if you have a new partner in the future, you'll feel more empowered to communicate what you enjoy and desire.

Menopause can be an opportunity to redefine what intimacy and pleasure mean to you. When we're younger, many of us have a pretty narrow script for sex. Midlife invites us to expand that script. Intimacy with a partner can include all kinds of erotic possibilities: kissing, cuddling, sensual massage, oral sex, mutual masturbation, taking a warm bath together, fantasizing together, or enjoying some steamy talk. Taking away the pressure to follow a certain set of "rules" can open up new avenues of pleasure. Some couples discover that outercourse (stimulation without penetration) actually leads to more orgasms or closeness. You might experiment with toys, erotic massage, reading erotica, or watching something arousing together. Trying new things can bring playfulness and fun, which can reignite your sexual energy.

One practical tip: if penetrative sex has been on pause for a while, you may need to ease back into it gradually. The vagina is a muscle-lined organ, and like any muscle, not using it can cause some tightening or initial discomfort when you start again. This is temporary. Take it slow, use plenty of lubricant, and consider some gentle stretching beforehand. You can even do a few pelvic floor relaxation exercises (for example, gently bear down as if to urinate, then relax) to help your muscles unclench.

You deserve pleasure, comfort, and closeness at every stage of life.

Intimacy is about pleasure and closeness, not any one specific act. For those in relationships, redefining intimacy can also mean focusing more on emotional closeness and non-sexual affection. Menopause can be a vulnerable time, and letting your partner see that vulnerability can deepen your connection. Sometimes, closeness and desire come back naturally when anxiety is reduced. You might set up date nights or simply start a habit of extended hugging and kissing each day without expecting it to lead to sex. Many couples find that their idea of a satisfying intimate evening broadens at this stage, maybe it's a candlelit back rub or cuddling and laughing in bed with a glass of wine and making out like teenagers. Let intimacy be anything that brings you together in a loving, present way.

Reclaiming Pleasure

Society has long sent the message that women over fifty aren't sexual or shouldn't be, which is pure nonsense. You are a full person with a range of appetites, and none of them define your worth. Your sexuality is personal and it's up to you. If we can bust the myth that menopause is the end of sensuality, women can reclaim this part of life with pride.

A healthy sex life is one that feels satisfying to you. You owe no one an explanation or justification for your desires (or lack of desire). If you've been embarrassed to talk about sex or to seek help for issues like vaginal dryness, know that menopause is finally becoming a more openly discussed topic. Doctors, especially menopause specialists, have truly heard it all. Nothing you're experiencing is "weird" or shameful. It's textbook menopause stuff, and there are solutions.

Reframing sexuality as vital and personal means recognizing that staying sexually active can be part of a vibrant, healthy life. Studies have even noted that women who continue to be intimate tend to report higher overall quality of life and emotional well-being. Orgasms release feel-good hormones like oxytocin and endorphins. These can boost your mood, relieve stress, and even help you sleep better. In this way, sexuality can be as much a wellness practice as it is a pleasure practice. On the other hand, if you choose to focus your energy in other areas (like relationships, creativity, or physical adventures), that's just as personal and valid. The common thread is that you are in charge of how you define and pursue pleasure.

Priya, 54, had always enjoyed a healthy sex life with her husband, but as she entered menopause, she noticed things were changing. Intercourse became painful, and her usual spark of desire was more like a flicker. She went from looking forward to their romantic nights to actively avoiding them. "I felt awful," Priya says. "I was not only dealing with hot flashes and mood swings, but now I worried my marriage would suffer. I kept thinking: Is this it? Am I just never going to want sex again?" She became so self-conscious about the pain that she started making excuses to skip intimacy, and her husband felt confused and rejected.

Finally, after a particularly tense weekend, Priya realized that avoiding the topic wasn't helping either of them. She sat down with her husband and told him everything, how her body had changed, how intercourse hurt due to dryness, how she missed the closeness but was afraid of the pain. To her relief, he didn't pull away or judge. He listened. Together, they came up with a plan. Priya visited her gynecologist, who confirmed she was experiencing vaginal atrophy. The doctor recommended a vaginal estrogen cream to use nightly for a few weeks and suggested a good silicone-based lubricant to use during sex. Priya also started doing daily pelvic floor exercises (she found a guided app to help).

The next time they were intimate, they took it slow. Priya used her new lubricant liberally and guided his hand to areas that felt good. They focused on plenty of foreplay, just enjoying each other without rushing. By the third or fourth try over the following weeks, Priya noticed a big improvement. The estrogen cream was doing its job. As the pain subsided, her interest in sex came back. She even found herself initiating intimacy for the first time in ages.

Do This Today

Choose one new strategy from this chapter to support your sexual health. For example:

- Buy a vaginal moisturizer and try using it this week.
- Add a few Kegel exercises into your morning routine.
- Explore self-pleasure as a way to reconnect with your body.

Pick one actionable step and give it a go. Your pleasure and joy are worth prioritizing.

Reflection

Ask yourself: "What is one step I can take to feel more comfortable and confident in my sexuality right now?"

Be honest and gentle as you consider this. It might be physical (trying a new remedy or exercise) or emotional (communicating a need to your partner or exploring what turns you on). Whatever you choose, remind yourself that you deserve care and pleasure.

Chapter 8
Biohacking for Well-Being

———

"The body will do what the body is designed to do if we stop interrupting it."

Dr. Sara Gottfried

———

Biohacking simply means using small, science-backed tweaks to optimize your well-being, based on feedback from your own body. For women in perimenopause and beyond, this can be a game-changer. Hormones shift, metabolism slows, recovery gets harder, but biohacking offers ways to restore balance and reawaken energy.

In your 40s and beyond, everything shifts, from your hormones to your recovery time and stress responses. What used to work, doesn't work quite the same. That's not a failure, it's feedback. Biohacking is about listening to your body, experimenting to see what helps, and customizing your self-care habits accordingly. Women's bodies are attuned to circadian rhythms, monthly cycles, and seasonal changes, so daily adjustments can produce big results over time.

Biohacking requires paying attention as your body quietly changes. These tiny tweaks remind you that you can nourish your energy, restore your focus, and protect your joy without overhauling your whole life. Some days, that might mean stepping outside into sunlight for five minutes instead of scrolling on your phone. Other days, it might mean taking magnesium at night or using cold therapy to reduce inflammation and lift your mood. These small adjustments can improve how you feel day to day, moment to moment.

How Biohacking Supports Your Hormones

Each biohack you introduce can act like a reset button for a particular hormone system:

Cortisol

This is your stress-response hormone. Breathwork helps recalibrate it, while cold exposure lowers baseline stress levels over time. Cutting out screens before bed and getting morning light can balance your natural cortisol rhythm, supporting better energy and sleep.

Estrogen

Estrogen plays a starring role in energy, skin, mood, and memory. As it declines, your body needs more support to metabolize and use it effectively. Liver-friendly hacks (like castor oil packs) and blood sugar-stabilizing habits (like eating protein or taking an apple cider vinegar supplement) can support estrogen without causing imbalance.

Progesterone

Known as the "chill hormone," progesterone promotes restful sleep. It often dips first in perimenopause, contributing to anxiety and insomnia. Magnesium, gentle fasting, and breathwork give your body signals to create more of this hormone.

Insulin

Insulin is highly responsive to lifestyle tweaks. High insulin leads to energy crashes, belly fat, and increased risk of diabetes. Daily movement, protein-rich meals, and even a tablespoon of apple cider vinegar before eating can improve insulin sensitivity and reduce those blood sugar roller coasters.

By gently and consistently targeting specific systems, biohacking becomes less about controlling your body and more about supporting it to do what it was designed to do all along.

Sarah was 47 when she realized she didn't recognize herself. She was a vibrant, energetic woman, but that had faded into someone who felt tired all the time, was easily overwhelmed, and disconnected from her body. Her mornings started with brain fog and a pounding heart, her energy dipped by noon, and her sleep felt like a nightly battle instead of rest. "I thought maybe this is just how it is now," she said. But then she began using simple biohacks.

She practiced expressive writing and breathwork whenever she felt anxious. She took a stress-relief supplement with L-theanine, GABA, and lemon balm. She started taking cold showers after workouts and made sure to stay hydrated and eat plenty of fresh fruits and vegetables. She added small tools like these, one by one. After two months, her energy was steadier, her moods were more balanced, and she finally felt like her vibrant self again.

Biohacks for Menopause Symptoms

It's not hard to introduce biohacks throughout your day to support your fluctuating energy. The following science-backed, real-life, friendly biohacks are tools, not strict rules. Start with one or two that feel manageable and try them for a few weeks to see how you feel.

Morning Light Exposure

Natural sunlight signals your brain to stop producing melatonin and start producing cortisol for natural energy. It resets your circadian rhythm, boosts serotonin, and improves sleep quality (Brown et al., 2022). Step outside for a few minutes early in the morning.

Hydration

Hydrate first thing. Drink 12–16 oz of water before coffee to rehydrate your body, support detox pathways, and help cortisol rise appropriately. Overnight we lose fluid, so water flushes toxins and kick-starts digestion. Continue to hydrate throughout the day to support your active system.

Protein-rich Breakfast

Protein reduces insulin spikes and supports lean muscle, especially after forty. Start your day with 25–30 g of protein to stabilize blood sugar, support muscle mass, and reduce cravings.

Cold Exposure

Cold triggers brown fat activity, boosts endorphins, and calms inflammation. Try cool showers or cold face dunks to activate your vagus nerve, support your metabolism, and lift your mood. Cold baths (or ice baths) can reduce inflammation and create an endorphin rush that leaves you feeling euphoric. They can be very brief and still effective! For beginners, aim for about five minutes.

Walking After Meals

A 10-minute walk after a meal lowers blood sugar, aids digestion, and supports metabolic health. Try walking after lunch, then hydrating and stretching before returning to work.

Gentle Fasting

Intermittent fasting helps reset digestion and balance hormones. For example, try fasting from 7 p.m. to 7 a.m. (a 12-hour window).

Digital Sunset

Turning off technology an hour or two before bedtime promotes deeper sleep.

Breathwork

Try box breathing to restore a sense of calm. Breathe in for 4 counts, hold for 4, breathe out for 4, and hold for 4. Repeat for a few cycles.

Dry Brushing

Before a shower, brush your skin with a dry brush using circular strokes toward your heart. This stimulates lymphatic drainage and blood flow.

Castor Oil Belly Packs

Castor oil packs are a natural remedy believed to help regulate hormones and reduce inflammation, bloating, and hot flashes. To try it: cut 3–4 strips of cotton fabric (about 10 x 12 inches). Soak them in castor oil and layer them to make a pack. Place the pack on your abdomen, cover it with plastic wrap, and then put a heating pad or hot water bottle on top. Rest with the heat on for 30–60 minutes.

Supplements

With a few intentional choices each day, you can reduce hot flashes, sleep better, and lift the brain fog. And with the right support, you can feel clear, strong, and fully yourself again. While hormone therapy is an option, many women look for natural, non-hormonal support to ease this transition. If you're interested in supplements, a few can help. Magnesium, electrolytes, and maca are popular choices. Some studies show that black cohosh reduces hot flash frequency (Leach & Moore, 2012). Omega-3s may improve blood vessel function related to hot flashes and night sweats, as well as improve mood (Lucas, 2011). Magnesium glycinate supports relaxation, regulates body temperature, aids sleep, reduces anxiety, and helps with hormonal balance. Vitamin E can reduce hot flash severity (Ziaei et al., 2007). Electrolytes help with dehydration and fatigue.

Adaptogenic herbs like maca and ashwagandha can support hormonal balance and energy. Collagen and protein powders can help muscle recovery and energy, and greens powders can boost your nutrient intake. It's best to focus on whole foods first, and then use supplements to target specific symptoms. When adding supplements, go slow: introduce one at a time and watch for side effects over a few weeks. Track any changes to see if the supplement is helping. And always check for interactions if you're on any medications.

Vitamin D3 + K2

Supports hormone balance, bone health, immunity, and mood.

Omega-3 fatty acids (EPA & DHA)

Support brain and heart health, reduce inflammation, and boost mood.

Ashwagandha

This adaptogen can lower cortisol and help with stress, balance hormones, ease hot flashes, reduce anxiety, and improve sleep.

Maca

This adaptogen may reduce hot flashes and mood swings, boost stamina and mental clarity, and support libido.

Rhodiola Rosea

This adaptogen can reduce fatigue, balance cortisol, sustain energy, and improve sleep and mood.

Moringa

Rich in antioxidants and micronutrients, it supports healthy blood sugar levels and may reduce hot flashes and improve sleep.

Magnesium

Often low in menopausal women, this mineral promotes muscle and nerve relaxation, and improves sleep and mood.

L-theanine

This amino acid promotes calm focus and helps with anxiety.

B-complex Vitamins

These are often low during menopause, which can cause fatigue and brain fog. B vitamins support cognitive function, mood, and energy.

Apple Cider Vinegar

Contains antioxidants, probiotics, and potassium. It may support gut health, stabilize blood sugar levels, and aid weight management. Try one teaspoon before meals or use it in salad dressings.

Electrolytes and Hydration

Hot flashes can cause electrolyte loss and worsen fatigue. Drink 2–3 liters of water each day and use electrolytes to boost hydration.

Coenzyme Q10 (CoQ10)

Studies show this antioxidant can support cognitive function and boost energy, mood, and sleep.

These supplements offer a powerful, evidence-informed approach to managing menopause. With the right mix of adaptogens, nutrients, hydration, light, and movement, you can ease symptoms, restore clarity, and feel strong again.

Symptom-Based Supplement Match

Poor Sleep	Magnesium glycinate, Ashwagandha, L-theanine
Hot Flashes/ Night Sweats	Vitamin E, Black Cohosh, Omega-3s
Brain Fog	Magnesium threonate, Omega-3s, B Vitamins, L-Theanine
Anxiety and Stress	Rhodiola, L-theanine, GABA
Low Energy	CoQ10, Iron (if deficient), Rhodiola
Mood Swings	Omega-3s, Vitamin D, Adaptogens
Libido/Sexual Dryness	Maca, Omega-3s, Vitamin E

Sumitra was 52 when the ground beneath her began to shift. She was a successful project manager, mother of two grown kids, and the go-to person in her friend group, and she always prided herself on her energy and clarity. But recently, she found herself staring blankly at her computer, unable to recall a password she had reset just the day before. Sleep became elusive. Her once dependable moods turned into a guessing game. The final straw came during a client presentation: mid-sentence, her face flushed and sweat beaded on her temples, and she couldn't remember what slide came next.

"I honestly thought I was losing it," Sumitra later shared. "I didn't recognize myself." Her doctor mentioned perimenopause and offered hormone therapy, but Sumitra wanted to explore natural options first. She started researching late into the night, scrolling through articles and podcasts and taking notes. Then she began experimenting. She added magnesium to her evening routine, sipped moringa tea in the afternoon, and dimmed the lights to help wind down before bed. The changes weren't overnight, but they were real. Her brain fog began to lift. She stopped dreading bedtime. Her energy, once scattered and fragile, started returning in quiet, steady waves. "I still have hard days, but I finally feel like I have tools that work with my body."

What Will Help Most Right Now?

Sometimes the hardest part of healing is knowing where to begin. Should you focus on sleep? Brain fog? Energy crashes? There's no perfect path, only the one that works best for you. Start simple with small changes, then go deeper if needed.

Hormonal shifts usually don't show up as a single symptom, they tend to travel in packs. Recognizing how symptoms cluster can help you see patterns and find solutions. Here are some of the most common symptom clusters:

Energy and Sleep Disruption

This cluster can include unrelenting fatigue, "crashing" fatigue (where you're moving at a normal pace and then suddenly feel completely exhausted), waking up multiple times at night, or feeling wired and tired at the same time. Fluctuating estrogen and progesterone levels disrupt sleep patterns by interfering with the body's ability to regulate temperature and mood (Gunter, 2021). For example, low progesterone levels which typically help you fall asleep, can make it harder to get deep, restorative sleep, leading to frequent night awakenings and poorer rest overall.

Cognitive Fog and Mood Swings

This includes difficulty concentrating, forgetfulness, anxiety, racing thoughts, sudden irritability, or feeling emotionally "off." These symptoms are often linked to changes in estrogen and serotonin levels, which affect mood and mental clarity. As estrogen dips, serotonin (the neurotransmitter that regulates mood) becomes less stable, which is why many women notice heightened irritability or depression during menopause (Brighten, 2019).

Weight and Metabolic Changes

This cluster can involve weight gain (especially around the abdomen), food cravings, bloating, and a frustrating resistance to weight loss despite diet or exercise. A decrease in estrogen can cause insulin resistance, making it harder to maintain a healthy weight. This is well documented: studies show that the decline in estrogen leads to fat redistributing more to the abdominal area, which is linked to an increased risk for heart disease and metabolic disorders like diabetes or thyroid issues (Greendale, 2017).

Temperature and Sensory Sensitivity

Symptoms like hot flashes, night sweats, and increased sensitivity to smells, noise, or lights. The hypothalamus, which regulates body temperature, is very sensitive to estrogen fluctuations, which explains these intense shifts. These sensations are often triggered by a drop in estrogen, which affects your body's ability to regulate temperature properly, resulting in hot flashes, night sweats, and even tingling skin (Haver, 2021).

Pain and Physical Sensitivity

This includes joint aches, muscle soreness, and increased inflammation or pain with exercise or inactivity. These symptoms often occur due to reduced estrogen levels. Less estrogen affects collagen production and increases inflammation. Lower estrogen can also lead to bone density loss, which contributes to aches and pains, especially in weight-bearing joints (Briden, 2021).

Remember, these symptoms aren't random, they contain important information about your body and how to find relief. When you identify which symptom clusters are affecting you, you can create targeted solutions. For example, stabilizing your blood sugar can help with both fatigue and mood swings. And practicing cooling strategies can manage hot flashes and improve sleep. As Dr. Aviva Romm notes in *Hormone Intelligence*, "When we track our symptoms as part of a bigger hormonal puzzle, we can stop guessing and start supporting our bodies intelligently." Knowledge is power, and recognizing patterns in your symptoms is the first step to reclaiming it.

If you feel fatigued, sluggish, or low energy...	• Begin your day with a glass of water with a pinch of sea salt and a squeeze of lemon.
	• Add an energy-boosting breakfast (for example, Greek yogurt with berries and seeds, or eggs with avocado toast). Consider taking a B-complex vitamin.
	• Take a brisk walk outdoors in the morning or do a few standing yoga poses to energize your body.
If your brain feels foggy or forgetful...	• Eat brain-friendly foods like walnuts, blueberries, eggs, and leafy greens. Consider adding a probiotic supplement.
	• Oxygenate your brain with a short yoga sequence (mountain pose, chair pose, crescent moon pose).
	• Take a break from technology in the evening and choose a creative activity like art, music, or gardening.
If you're irritable, moody, or anxious more often...	• Practice alternate nostril breathing.
	• Balance blood sugar by including protein plus healthy fat at each meal (for example, salmon, quinoa, greens).
	• Spend a few minutes walking outdoors and listening to the environment.

If you're struggling with hot flashes or poor sleep...	• Start with good sleep hygiene, vagus nerve stimulation, relaxation techniques, and supportive nutrition/supplements.
	• Keep your bedroom cool, wear breathable cotton, and cut down on alcohol and caffeine.
	• Hold an ice pack against the side of your neck (below your ears) to stimulate the vagus nerve and relax your nervous system.
	• Eat foods with phytoestrogens like flaxseeds, tofu, or hummus. Consider supplements like magnesium glycinate and evening primrose oil.
If you feel uninspired, unmotivated, or disconnected...	• Spend time in nature, and nurture connection.
	• Unplug from social media to reconnect with yourself.
	• Do something playful every day like doodle, sing, play fetch with your dog.
	• Add colorful fruits and vegetables to your meals (like bell peppers, berries, spinach).

If your weight is creeping up despite healthy habits...	• Prioritize protein and fiber in your diet.
	• Avoid late-night snacking. Try a 12-hour eating window (for example, finish dinner by 7 p.m. and have breakfast after 7 a.m.).
	• Add strength training exercises: use dumbbells or a medicine ball and include bodyweight moves like wall push-ups or squats.
	• Try a loving kindness meditation: begin by offering yourself kind wishes (e.g., "May I be safe, may I be happy, may I be healthy, may I be free."). Then offer the same blessings to all beings.

Do This Today

Pick one biohack from this chapter to experiment with. Stick with it for two weeks and track how you feel. Pay attention to your sleep quality, mood, and energy levels, as well as how easy it is to maintain the habit.

Reflection

Ask yourself: "Which part of my day feels rushed or chaotic? What would bring peace to that moment and help me feel more grounded? How can I make it as easy as possible for myself?"

Chapter 9
The 28-Day Menopause Reset Challenge

Hopefully, by now you've started to use what you've been learning to make some positive changes to your daily routine. This final part of the book encourages you to create a simple daily plan to help you explore what works for your unique needs and put some healthy new habits into action.

This 28-Day Reset Challenge isn't a boot camp. There's no punishment for missing a day. It's a compassionate commitment to yourself, designed to build momentum, energy, and confidence through stackable habits and simple, repeatable actions. Each week focuses on a new theme, from movement to mindset, and you'll only need ten minutes a day. Science shows that habit formation thrives when we track progress, stay curious, and adapt our strategies (Clear, 2018). By using the following printables, you'll continue tuning into your body, learning what works, and stacking small wins that lead to big shifts.

If you track your progress every day, you will become aware of what is helping, and what isn't. Psychiatrist and mindfulness researcher, Dr. Daniel Siegel says, "When you name it, you tame it." When you jot down what you're doing and how you're feeling, you start to notice connections. What lifts you up, what drains you, and how your energy, mood, and focus change depending on what you are doing, how you are eating, and what conditions might be changing. These small reflections strengthen your focus and attention, and that's where real transformation begins.

Try to pay attention to how you feel mentally and physically, as well as what nutrition, supplements, movement, or mindfulness activities you include in each day. When you track your mood, try to be as specific as possible. Do you feel calm, happy, numb, full of rage, unfocused? Try to notice patterns, triggers, helpful tools, or anything else that seems potentially connected.

Over time, you'll spot predictable rhythms, notice how nutrition or stress affects your mood, and develop better emotional resilience.

You can use the daily trackers to help you capture all of the layers of helpful details, to see if any patterns begin to emerge.

Bonus Support for Your 28-Day Reset

To make your reset easier, I've included a full **10 Minute Menopause Toolkit** with extra resources you can use anytime:

- 28-Day Reset Printouts and Trackers
- Quick-Start 5-Ingredient Meal Plans
- Symptom and Progress Trackers
- Wall Pilates and Somatic Flows
- Affirmations, Positivity Tools and CBT Worksheets
- And More

Access your toolkit here:

https://menopause.habitkind.store/bonus

Or simply scan the QR code

SCAN ME

Think of these as your bonus companions, keeping you supported every step of the way.

Monthly Menopause Symptom Tracker

This tracker is designed to help you become more aware of your body's patterns throughout the month. By logging your symptoms daily, you'll begin to see trends, identify potential triggers, and better prepare for what your body needs. This tool can also be helpful to share with your healthcare provider for more personalized care.

To begin tracking your symptoms, download and print your tracker using this link or copy the format into your journal.

Each evening, take a moment to review the symptoms listed. For any symptom you experienced that day, mark it by assigning an intensity rating (1-5). You can also use the 'Notes' section to jot down any observations.

DAYS	1	2	3	4	5	6	7	8	9	10	11	12	13	14	15	16	17	18	19	20	21	22	23	24	25	26	27	28
Hot Flashes																												
Bloating																												
Brain Fog																												
Racing Thoughts																												
Weight Gain																												
Night Sweats																												
Crashing Fatigue																												
Fatigue																												
Joint Pain																												
Thinning Hair																												
Anxiety																												
Mood Swings																												
Sleep Disturbances																												
Other symptoms																												

Week 1 Movement and Morning Mojo

*The way you start your day determines how
well you live your day.*
Robin Sharma

Regular physical activity is associated with improved vasomotor symptoms, mood, and sleep in menopausal women (Elavsky & McAuley, 2007).

	10-Minutes to Embrace Movement	☑ Done
Day 1	Take a walk outside— bonus if it's in sunlight.	
Day 2	Do a gentle stretching routine.	
Day 3	Do something playful (like dancing or singing).	
Day 4	Try "Box Breathing" + some spinal twists.	
Day 5	Do a short Wall Pilates sequence.	
Day 6	Practice a weight resistance routine.	
Day 7	Take a barefoot walk outdoors to ground yourself & be in your body.	

Week 2 Food and Fuel

Let food be thy medicine and medicine be thy food.
Hippocrates

Every time you eat, it's an opportunity to nourish your body. The right foods help balance blood sugar, reduce inflammation, and give you more energy.

	10-Minute Reset Action	☑ **Done**
Day 8	Make a colorful plate: add three or more different veggies to one meal.	
Day 9	Prep a hormone-friendly snack: nuts, seeds, fruit.	
Day 10	Drink a glass of lemon water before your morning coffee.	
Day 11	Swap sugar for cinnamon, vanilla, or ginger in your tea or oatmeal.	
Day 12	Try a new leafy green (arugula, dandelion, kale, etc.).	
Day 13	Plan three protein-rich meals for next week.	
Day 14	Eat mindfully: no distractions, chew slowly, taste your food.	

Week 3 Recovery and Calm

Almost everything will work again if you unplug it for a few minutes... including you.
Anne Lamott

Rest is not a luxury, it's a biological necessity. Recovery habits help lower cortisol, soothe your nervous system, and build resilience.

	10-Minute Reset Action	☑ Done
Day 15	Do a 10-minute meditation.	
Day 16	Take a hot bath or foot soak with Epsom salts.	
Day 17	Try legs-up-the-wall pose or pigeon pose. Breathe deeply.	
Day 18	Write down three things you feel grateful for.	
Day 19	Read or journal in a quiet space.	
Day 20	Do absolutely nothing. Let yourself just be.	
Day 21	Step outside, breathe in fresh air, and stretch to the sky.	

Week 4 Sleep and Mindset

Sleep is the best meditation.
Dalai Lama

Good sleep restores your body, balances hormones, and sharpens focus. A clear mindset helps you handle stress and stay resilient.

	10-Minute Reset Action	**☑ Done**
Day 22	Set a digital sunset: no screens one hour before bed.	
Day 23	Focus on your evening wind-down ritual.	
Day 24	Write down one worry. Then write: "I release this."	
Day 25	Improve your bedroom environment: eye mask, blackout curtains, fan, etc.	
Day 26	Prep a magnesium-rich snack: banana, almonds, or seeds.	
Day 27	Try a yoga nidra or yin yoga session.	
Day 28	Journal: "How have I changed over the last 28 days?"	

Find Your Rhythm of Care

You've made it. You've learned about the science of hormones, and you've become more deeply aware of what you need to feel better. You've shown up for yourself, and now, it's time to carry that momentum forward by continuing to find your rhythm of care, every day. It's about staying present for yourself, recognizing when you need a little extra support, and continuing to learn how to adapt to your changing needs.

You've already taken the most important step to feeling better: paying attention. There will be days that feel off. There may be relapses, forgetfulness, or nights of poor sleep. But what matters isn't perfection, it's presence. Your willingness to keep showing up for yourself, even in 10-minute doses, is everything. Now, take this toolkit and adapt it to what helps you most.

Thousands of women are quietly rewriting the rules of midlife. You are part of that quiet revolution. So, start where you are. Use what you have. Do what you can. Then watch what shifts. You just need one small bit of relief at a time to remind your body and your mind what it feels like to thrive.

References

Abbasi, B. et al. (2012). The effect of magnesium supplementation on primary insomnia in elderly: A double blind placebo controlled clinical trial. National Research in Medical Sciences. Retrieved from: https://pmc.ncbi.nlm.nih.gov/articles/PMC3703169/

Baumeister, R. F. et al. (1998). Ego depletion. Journal of Personality and Social Psychology. https://doi.org/10.1037/0022 3514.74.5.1252

Bianchi, V. E. et al. (2021). The role of androgens in women's health and wellbeing. Pharmacological Research.

Borst, S. et al. (2001). Effects of resistance training on insulin like growth factor I and IGF binding proteins. Medicine and Science in Sports and Exercise.

Brizendine, L. (2006). The Female Brain. Morgan Road Books.

Briden, L. (2021). Hormone Repair Manual. Pan Macmillan.

Brighten, J. (2023). Is This Normal? Judgment-free Straight Talk About Your Body. HarperOne.

Brown, TM et al. (2022). Recommendations for daytime, evening, and nighttime indoor light exposure to best support physiology, sleep, and wakefulness in healthy adults. PLOS Biology. https://journals.plos.org/plosbiology/article?id=10.1371%2Fjournal.pbio.3001571&

Bulman, A. et al. (2025). The effects of L theanine consumption on sleep outcomes: A systematic review and meta analysis. Science Direct. https://www.sciencedirect.com/science/article/pii/S1087079225000292

Capel Alcaraz, A. M. et al.(2023). The efficacy of strength exercises for reducing the symptoms of menopause. Journal of Clinical Medicine.

Carpenter, J. et al. (2018). Cognitive behavioral therapy for anxiety and related disorders: A meta analysis of randomized placebo controlled trials. National Library of Medicine. https://pubmed.ncbi.nlm.nih.gov/29451967/

Chellew, K. et al. (2015). The effect of progressive muscle relaxation on daily cortisol secretion. National Library of Medicine. https://pubmed.ncbi.nlm.nih.gov/26130387/

Colberg, S. R. et al. (2016). Physical activity/exercise and diabetes. National Library of Medicine. https://pubmed.ncbi.nlm.nih.gov/27926890/

Collins, B. C. et al. (2019). Aging of the musculoskeletal system. ScienceDirect Journals and Books. https://www.sciencedirect.com/science/article/abs/pii/S8756328219301206

Clear, J. (2018). Atomic Habits. Avery.

Dalton Smith, S.(2017). Sacred Rest. FaithWords.

Davis, S. R. et al. (2015). Menopause. Nature Reviews Disease Primers. https://www.nature.com/articles/nrdp20154

Doidge, N. (2007). The Brain That Changes Itself. Viking.

Dreisoerner, A. et al. (2021). Self soothing touch and being hugged reduce cortisol responses to stress: a randomized controlled trial on stress, physical touch, and social identity. National Library of Medicine . https://pubmed.ncbi.nlm.nih.gov/35757667/

Duhigg, C. (2012). The Power of Habit. Random House.

Davis, S. R., et al. (2012). Understanding weight gain at menopause. Climacteric. https://doi.org/10.3109/13697137.2012.707385

Elavsky, S. and E. McAuley (2007). Physical activity and mental health outcomes during menopause: A randomized controlled trial. Annals of Behavioral Medicine. https://doi.org/10.1007/BF02879894

Esther, P. (2006). Mating in Captivity. Harper Collins.

Farshbaf Khalili, A. et al. (2020). The effect of oral capsule of curcumin and vitamin E on the hot flashes and anxiety in postmenopausal women: A triple blind randomised controlled trial. Complementary Therapies in Medicine

Fogg, B. J. (2019). Tiny Habits. Houghton Mifflin Harcourt.

Freeman, E. W. et al. (2015). Poor sleep in relation to natural menopause: a population based 14 year follow up of midlife women. https://pubmed.ncbi.nlm.nih.gov/25549066/

Freeman, E. W. & K. Sherif. (2007). Prevalence of hot flashes and night sweats around the world. Climacteric. https://pubmed.ncbi.nlm.nih.gov/25549066/

Gasnick, K. (2024). Exercises That Worsen Osteoarthritis. Very Well Health. https://www.verywellhealth.com/exercises that make osteoarthritis worse 5215265?utm_source

Gatenby, C. & P. Simpson. (2024). Menopause. Best Practice & Research Clinical Endocrinology & Metabolism.

Goins, S. (2023). Managing sleep during menopause. Mayo Clinic Minute. https://newsnetwork.mayoclinic.org/discussion/mayo clinic minute managing sleep during menopause/

Gottfried, S. (2013). The Hormone Cure. Scribner.

Gottfried, S. Women, Food, and Hormones. Mariner Book.00s, 2021.

Greendale, GA, et al. (2023). Cardiometabolic shifts during menopause. The Lancet Diabetes & Endocrinology.

Gunter, J. The Menopause Manifesto. Kensington Books, 2013.

Haghayegh, S., et al. (2019). Before-bedtime passive body heating by warm shower or bath to improve sleep: A systematic review and meta-analysis. Sleep Medicine Reviews, 46. https://doi.org/10.1016/j.smrv.2019.04.008

Hansen, M. (2021). Sex hormonal effects on tendons and ligaments in fascia in sport and movement. Handspring Publishing Limited.

Haver, M. C. (2023). The Galveston Diet. Rodale Books.

Ho, G. et al. (2023). Strength training is associated with less knee osteoarthritis: data from the osteoarthritis initiative. American College of Rheumatology. https://acrjournals.onlinelibrary.wiley.com/doi/10.1002/art.42732?

Huffington, A. (2017). The Sleep Revolution. Penguin Random House

Hurtado, M. D. et al. (2024). Weight gain in midlife women. Current Obesity Reports.

Hyman, M. (2021). The Pegan Diet. Little Brown Spark.

Kandiah, J. (2010). An exploratory study on perceived relationship of alcohol, caffeine, and physical activity on hot flashes in menopausal women. ResearchGate. Retrieved from: https://www.researchgate.net/publication/274413314_An_exploratory_study_on_perceived_relationship_of_alcohol_caffeine_and_physical_activity_on_hot_flashes_in_menopausal_women

Kaushal, A., et al. (2017). Increasing physical activity through principles of habit formation in new gym members: a randomized controlled trial. National Library of Medicine. https://pubmed.ncbi.nlm.nih.gov/28188586/

Kelley, D. E. et al. (2002). Muscle triglyceride and insulin resistance. Annual Review of Nutrition. https://www.deepdyve.com/lp/annual reviews/muscle triglyceride and insulin resistance kMy7XL0hVB

Kolata, G. (2021). What we think to know about metabolism may be wrong. International New York Times.

Kravitz, H. M. and H. Joffe. (2011). Sleep during the perimenopause. Obstetrics and Gynecology Clinics.

Khorrami N. (2020). Gratitude helps minimize feelings of stress. Psychology Today. https://www.psychologytoday.com/us/blog/comfort gratitude/202007/gratitude helps minimize feelings stress?

Laborde, S. et al (2022). Effects of voluntary slow breathing on heart rate and heart rate variability: a systematic review and a meta analysis. National Library of Medicine. https://pubmed.ncbi.nlm.nih.gov/35623448/

LePera, N. (2021) How to Do the Work. Harper Wave.

Leach, M. J. and V. Moore. (2012). Black cohosh for menopausal symptoms. Cochrane Database of Systematic Reviews. https://pubmed.ncbi.nlm.nih.gov/22972105/

Leidy, H. J. et al. (2015). The role of protein in weight loss and maintenance. The American

Journal of Clinical Nutrition.

Lemoine, P. et al. (2011). Prolonged release melatonin for insomnia An open label long term study of efficacy, safety, and withdrawal. Therapeutic and Clinical Risk Management.

Li, W. (2023). Eat to Beat Your Diet. Random House.

Long periods of sedentary behavior may increase cardiovascular risk in older women (2019). National Health Institute. https://www.nih.gov/news events/news releases/long periods sedentary behavior may increase cardiovascular risk older women?

Lucas, M. et al. (2011). Dietary intake of n 3 and n 6 fatty acids and the risk of clinical depression in women: a 10 y prospective follow up study. National Library of Medicine. https://pubmed.ncbi.nlm.nih.gov/21471279/

Lyon, G. (2020). Muscle centric medicine. Retrieved from https://drgabriellelyon.com

Lyon, G. (2023). Forever Strong. Atria Books.

Manson, J. E. et al. (2020). Vitamin D, omega 3s, and primary prevention of cardiovascular disease and cancer. The New England Journal of Medicine. https://pubmed.ncbi.nlm.nih.gov/31895658/

Meraglia, T. (2014). The Hormone Secret. Atria Books.

Moline, M. L. et al. (2003). Sleep in women across the life cycle from adulthood through menopause. Sleep Medicine Reviews.

Nagoski, E. (2025). Come Together. Penguin Random House.

Nappi, R. E. (2022). The 2022 hormone therapy position statement of The North American Menopause Society: no news is good news. The Lancet Diabetes & Endocrinology.

National Institutes of Health. (2023). Menopause: Overview. https://medlineplus.gov/menopause.html

Nelson, M. E. et al. (2007). Physical activity and public health in older adults. Medicine & Science in Sports & Exercise. https://doi.org/10.1249/mss.0b013e3180616a

Northrup, C. (2021). The Wisdom of Menopause. Bantam.

North American Menopause Society. (2022). The Menopause Guidebook (10th ed.).

North American Menopause Society. (2021). Managing Menopause. https://doi.org/10.1016/j.jmm.2020.10.001

Office of Dietary Supplements, NIH. (2024). Dietary Supplement Fact Sheets. https://ods.od.nih.gov/factsheets/list all/

Orsatti, F. L. et al. (2022). Heterogeneity in resistance training induced muscle strength responses is associated with training frequency and insulin resistance in postmenopausal women. Experimental Gerontology.

Paterson, D. H. and D. E. Warburton. (2010). Physical activity and functional limitations in older adults. International Journal Behavioral Nutrition and Physical Activity. https://ijbnpa.biomedcentral.com/articles/10.1186/1479 5868 7 38

Pelz, M. (2023). Fast like a girl. Hay House Inc.

Prior, J. C. (2011). Progesterone for symptom control during perimenopause. Women's Health. 6.5 (2010): 681 695. https://pubmed.ncbi.nlm.nih.gov/24753856/

Reed, D. L. and W. P. Sacco. (2016). Measuring sleep efficiency. Sleep Health. https://pubmed.ncbi.nlm.nih.gov/26194727/

Robertson, R. P. and J. S. Harmon. (2020). Pancreatic islet beta cell and oxidative stress. Diabetes, Obesity and Metabolism. https://pubmed.ncbi.nlm.nih.gov/17433304/

Romm, A. (2021). Hormone intelligence. HarperOne.

Rubin, G. (2015). Better Than Before. Crown Publishing Group. Columbia University Irving Medical Center. (2023). Rx for prolonged sitting: s five minute stroll every half hour. https://www.cuimc.columbia.edu/news/rx prolonged sitting five minute stroll every half hour?

Ryan, A. S. et al. (1996). Resistive training increases insulin action in postmenopausal women. The Journals of Gerontology Series A: Biological Sciences and Medical Sciences.

Sarmento, A. et al (2021). Genitourinary syndrome of menopause: epidemiology, physiopathology, clinical manifestation and diagnostic. Frontiers in Reproductive Health. https://www.frontiersin.org/journals/reproductive health/articles/10.3389/frph.2021.779398/full?utm_source

Scavello, I. et al. (2019). Sexual health in menopause. National Library of Medicine. https://pmc.ncbi.nlm.nih.gov/articles/PMC6780739/?

Sengupta, P. (2012). Health impacts of yoga and pranayama. International Journal of Preventive Medicine.

Shapcott E. (2024). Joint and muscle pain in perimenopausal women: causes, presentation, and treatment. Sheddon Physiotherapy and Sports Clinic Oakville https://www.sheddonphysio.com/joint and muscle pain in perimenopausal women causes presentation and treatment/

Shaw, G. (2017). The role of magnesium in managing menopause fatigue. Journal of Clinical Endocrinology & Metabolism. https://doi.org/10.1210/jc.2017 0166

Siegel, D. J. and T. P. Bryson (2011). The Whole Brain Child. Delacorte.

Sims, S. (2020). Roar. Rodale Books.

Sims, S. (2022). Next Level. Rodale Books.

Sinek, S. (2009). Start With Why. Portfolio.

Srivastava, N. et al. (2010). Standardization of Sterilization Protocol for Micropropagation of Aconitum heterophyllum An Endangered Medicinal Herb. Scientific Research. Retrieved from: https://www.scirp.org/reference/referencespapers?referenceid=2152826

St Onge, M. P. et al. (2016). Sleep and duration on energy balance. Current Nutrition Reports. https://www.researchgate.net/publication/308609140

Szeliga, A. et al. (2021). Gut microbiota in menopause. Menopause Review.

Taavoni, S. et al. (2020). 2363 Effect Of Valerian On Sleep Quality In Menopausal Women: a Randomized Placebo Controlled Clinical Trial. Cambridge University Press.

Tandon, V. R. et al. (2022). Menopause and sleep disorders. Journal of Mid Life Health.

Thurston, R. et al. (2013). Adipokines, adiposity, and vasomotor symptoms during the menopause transition: findings from the Study of Women's Health Across the Nation. National Library of Medicine. https://pubmed.ncbi.nlm.nih.gov/23755948/

Tolle, E. (2004). The Power of Now. New World Library.

Vitti, A. (2020). In the FLO. HarperOne.

Vohs, K. D. et al. (2014). Making choices impairs subsequent self control. Journal of Personality and Social Psychology.

Walker, M. (2017). Why We Sleep: Unlocking the Power of Sleep and Dreams.

Women's Mental Health Consortium (2019). The Women's Guide to Overcoming Insomnia: Get a Good Night's Sleep Without Relying on Medication. Retrieved: https://wmhcny.org/s/cbt for insomnia not just sleep hygiene?

Wurtman, R. J. et al.. (2003). Precursor control of neurotransmitter synthesis. Pharmacological Reviews.

Yang, J. M. et al. (2022). Effects of resistance training on body composition and physical function in elderly patients with osteosarcopenic obesity.Archives of Osteoporosis.

Yano, J. M. et al. (2015). Indigenous bacteria from the gut microbiota regulate host serotonin biosynthesis. National Library of Medicine. https://pubmed.ncbi.nlm.nih.gov/25860609/

Yoh, K., et al. (2023). Roles of estrogen, estrogen receptors, and estrogen related receptors in skeletal muscle. International Journal of Molecular Sciences.

Zhao, M. et al. (2019). Beneficial associations of low and large doses of leisure time physical activity on risk of mortality: a national cohort study of US adults aged 40 85 years. National Library of Medicine. https://pubmed.ncbi.nlm.nih.gov/30890520

Ziaei, S. et al. (2007). The effect of vitamin E on hot flashes in menopausal women. Gynecologic and Obstetric Investigation. https://pubmed.ncbi.nlm.nih.gov/17664882/

Thank You Bonus

Your reset doesn't stop here. As part of your plan, you get access to a full 10-Minute Menopause Toolkit with:

- 28-Day Reset Printouts and Trackers
- Affirmation Cards for Daily Encouragement
- CBT and Positivity Workbooks for Mindset Support
- 5-Ingredient Sweet and Savory Recipes with Shopping Lists
- Follow-Along Somatic Practices and Wall Pilates Videos
- And More

Access your toolkit here:

https://menopause.habitkind.store/bonus

SCAN ME

Or simply scan the QR code to download everything instantly

A simple plan to support your body and mind in just 10 minutes a day.

www.ingramcontent.com/pod-product-compliance
Lightning Source LLC
Chambersburg PA
CBHW031520270326
41930CB00006B/453